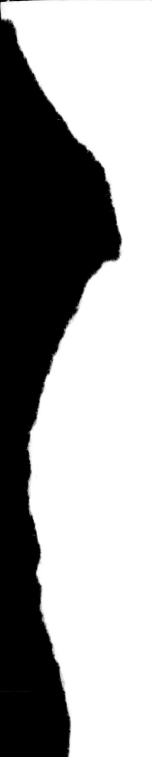

BONNIE BUXTO

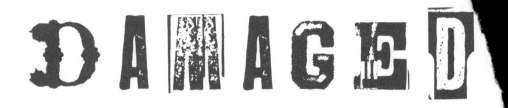

DAMAGED

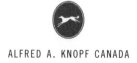

ALFRED A. KNOPF CANADA

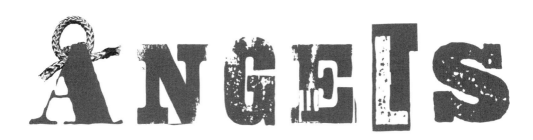

ANGELS

A Mother Discovers the Terrible Cost
of Alcohol in Pregnancy

PUBLISHED BY ALFRED A. KNOPF CANADA

Copyright © 2004 Bonnie Buxton

National Library of Canada Cataloguing in Publication

Buxton, Bonnie

Damaged angels : a mother discovers the terrible cost of alcohol in pregnancy / Bonnie Buxton.

Includes bibliographical references and index.

ISBN 0-676-97638-7

1. Fetal alcohol syndrome. 2. Children of prenatal alcohol abuse.

I. Title.

RG629.F45B89 2004   618.3'268   C2003-905816-6

First Edition

www.randomhouse.ca

Text design: Carla Kean

Printed and bound in Canada

10 9 8 7 6 5 4 3 2 1

In loving memory of my parents,
Dr. Earl William Buxton and Dorothy Lee Buxton,
and my friend Keitha Dion McLean

And in hope that
in Kenneth and Victoria
the cycle has been forever broken

Cherish pity, lest you drive an angel from your door.

—WILLIAM BLAKE, "HOLY THURSDAY"

CONTENTS

Three-year-old Colette was a "golden child"—bright, determined, beautiful and funny. Who could resist? We fought to adopt her, not knowing it would be only the first of many battles for her—and with her.

When our delightful preschooler morphed into a delinquent street kid, we sought a reason behind her learning and behaviour problems. What had we done wrong? A series of social workers, psychiatrists and therapists couldn't provide an answer.

We discovered that the preventable birth defect that permanently damages 1 percent of infants in the industrialized world is now known as fetal alcohol spectrum disorder (FASD). Like an iceberg, most of it lurks below the surface.

During their lifetimes, about 40 percent of individuals with FASD will experience "trouble with the law," and about 25 percent of incarcerated offenders have FASD. People with FASD are also more likely to be victims of crime. Here are some crime stories in which FASD may play an invisible role.

Alcoholism is the child of despair in aboriginal communities everywhere, in slums and tenements in North America and the United Kingdom, in shantytowns in the Caribbean, Africa and South America, throughout the countries of the former Soviet Union—and in upper-class families throughout the world. Meet five international FASD fighters.

Certain parents have eyes that dance when they talk about their children with FASD—children who have become poets, artists, dancers, musicians, athletes or, simply, fine human beings. These Superparents inspire the rest of us with their patience, wisdom and humour.

Like childbirth fever, smallpox and polio, FASD can be beaten—but money alone is not enough. The task requires awareness of the effects of prenatal alcohol, by top members of government as well as individual members of the community, along with the application of strategies developed over the past three decades.

FOREWORD

My first meeting with Bonnie Buxton was a total surprise. She dashed across the room, put her arms around me and told me that I was her hero! On reflection, I realized that Bonnie and her husband, Brian Philcox, along with countless other parents, grandparents and care-givers of children affected with fetal alcohol spectrum disorder (FASD) are the real heroes. Bonnie's passionate portrayal of her family's journey in *Damaged Angels* tells of the pervasive effects of prenatal alcohol exposure through their own struggle for understanding of their daughter Colette's disability. Their story is repeated too often in this country and worldwide.

In *Damaged Angels* we learn about how ill-equipped many professionals are to diagnose and treat children with a preventable disorder that affects nearly 1% of our population. Only a fraction of affected children present with identifiable facial features. Most children's impairments are invisible, but they are profoundly challenged, especially in areas of social skills and common sense. These are the children who "pass the tests but fail life." We learn about the lack of resources in the community, and the profound frustration experienced by parents of children and adolescents with FASD. We learn about the heart-wrenching experiences that parents are faced with on a daily basis in trying to make the system and our society respond to and understand their children and their needs. We also learn of events that give us hope. Bonnie gives us glimpses of how much can be achieved through support networks, and we witness the perseverance of the children and families in spite of seemingly insurmountable adversity.

I believe attitudes are changing for the better: there is now more government funding for FASD education, prevention, diagnosis, screening and intervention programs, but we still have a long way to go. Professionals dealing with pregnant women caught up in addiction, or lifestyles that involve alcohol and drug use, now realize more than ever that they are dealing with two patients, the expectant mother and the unborn child. Both are in need of specialized assistance and care. Mothers are often portrayed as the villains—but in truth, both the mother and the unborn child are often the victims of a sometimes complex and chaotic social environment. They often don't have the support they need from their partner or family to properly care for themselves during pregnancy. In recent years, social service workers, child protection workers and health care providers have awakened to the revelation that practical, genuine care, counselling and treatment for the mother will improve the outcome for the child, and can lead to the prevention of alcohol use in subsequent pregnancies. Several mentoring programs in our country such as Stop FAS in Manitoba and First Steps in Alberta have proven to be successful.

There has also been a change in our attitude towards the adoptive parents of affected children. In the past, professionals tended to blame, or were perceived to blame the parents for being poor caregivers, failing their children and contributing to the child's out-of-control behaviour. We now recognize that this behaviour is often the result of brain damage, and is not controllable through traditional discipline and child-rearing practices. Changing attitudes and using intervention techniques to fit the child's disability and learning style can benefit the well-being of the child and also help caregivers and teachers respond more effectively.

Health economists and social policy makers now know that for every dollar spent on prevention, there can be a future saving of five to seven dollars. The lifetime cost for care of an individual with FASD can exceed one million dollars. Governments should use every means possible to educate the public and those at risk about the adverse and profound effects of prenatal alcohol exposure. The message needs to be clear and unambiguous—no alcohol in pregnancy is best. Warning labels on alcoholic beverages alerting consumers to the dangers of alcohol in pregnancy would offer a strong symbolic message to the public. Research reveals that there is probably no threshold for effects of alcohol on the fetal brain, but the effects are based on a dose response. Mild social drinking (as little as an average of one alcoholic beverage per week) has been associated with measurable adverse effects on children's behaviour and attention spans later on.

Governments need to spend more money on research as well as the proper evaluation of prevention, intervention, education and training programs. They need to spend more on the development of multidisciplinary diagnostic and treatment clinics that can reach the communities at greatest risk. More funding needs to be directed to job training programs, prevention and addiction treatment programs. Reducing the secondary disabilities in an individual with FASD will benefit everyone. Many alcohol-affected adults have few supports and find themselves on the fringes of society—without an adequate education they are unable to obtain or hold gainful employment and find themselves living in poverty or on the streets. Some turn to crime out of a simple need to survive, but often it is because of their gullibility and eagerness to please others who sometimes use them for their own sinister purposes.

Many individuals with FASD are trapped in our prison system: they may repeatedly return to jail because they continually break rules and avoid restrictions that they do not and cannot understand. Finding and training mentors, providing housing and developing appropriate job training programs for adults with FASD must be a higher priority for social services in our communities.

So where will the money come from for these programs and supports? Should the primary responsibility fall to the taxpayer? What about the alcohol industry's moral obligation to pay some of these costs? Although they have taken some initiatives, their contributions fall far short of the need.

Bonnie has written an extraordinary, lucid and gripping account of parents living with an alcohol-affected child from infancy into adulthood. She shows us how a diagnosis of FASD results in a paradigm shift in everyone's attitude towards the person affected—from seeing a person who is mean, defiant, lazy and uncooperative to seeing a person with a neurological disability who needs a specialized approach to care, education and treatment. Her analysis of the current state of supports for individuals with FASD is a clarion call to the nation. She provides the reader with sound advice on the need for our governments and our communities to take immediate action.

Bonnie writes with authority gained from her journey with Colette and her gathering of many other families' experiences in Canada and abroad. Her professional training and experience as a journalist have given her the skills to search further—she has met, interviewed and learned from the most expert practitioners in the field of FASD. I predict that Bonnie Buxton's *Damaged Angels* will surpass the phenomenal impact of Michael Dorris's award-winning memoir, *The Broken Cord*. I promise that reading *Damaged Angels* will be a moving experience, and at the same time the book will help readers understand more fully the challenges and truths that we face concerning the plight of our children and adults with FASD.

Dr. Ab Chudley
December 2003

Dr. Albert E. (Ab) Chudley is a pediatrician, medical geneticist and clinician researcher in Winnipeg and a professor at the University of Manitoba. He has over twenty-five years of experience in diagnosing, treating and counselling FASD children, adults and their families. In May 2000 Dr. Chudley was appointed a member on Health Canada's National Advisory Committee on FASD.

ACKNOWLEDGMENTS

This book could not have been written without a world of extraordinary people, contributing their experience and knowledge. It also could not have been written without the more than thirty years of research at University of Washington—particularly the team responsible for the original *Lancet* study in 1973, and the continuing work for more than three decades by Ann Streissguth, Ph.D., and Dr. Sterling Clarren. Without this critically important research and outreach, our family—and countless others—would still be struggling for answers to our children's puzzling problems.

Nor would this book have been possible without the compassion of the pediatric geneticist Dr. Ab Chudley of Winnipeg, Manitoba, who responded to my desperate letter in the fall of 1997 and confirmed what in my heart I already knew: that our daughter's learning and behaviour problems were related to alcohol damage she suffered before she was born. Dr. Chudley has continued to be supportive, and for his unfailing help I am truly grateful. Thank you, Dr. Kathy Jones, for connecting me with Dr. Chudley, for participating in this book and for your continuing friendship and humour.

I could not have written it without the FASlink listserv, created in 1996 by the Canadian Centre for Substance Abuse, funded by Health Canada. Since 1999, FASlink has been operated by Bruce Ritchie of Sarnia, Ontario, who as a hardworking volunteer has archived more than 80,000 e-mail posts from parents and professionals, creating the world's most valuable source of first-hand information about the lives of individuals with FASD, and their families.

Special thanks to my agent, Beverley Slopen, for her strong support. I'm grateful to Diane Martin, publisher and editor at Knopf Canada for her keen enthusiasm and gentle nurturing; to trade paperback publisher Marion Garner for supporting publication of this edition; and to managing editor Deirdre Molina and editorial assistant Angelika Glover for their endless patience.

Thank you, Stevie Cameron, for answering my 1997 query to *Elm Street* magazine and giving me the opportunity to write the article "Society's Child" in my own voice. Thank you, Terry Palmer, for urging me to write this book.

Damaged Angels is richer because of the long-term help of Stephen Neafcy, a survivor of FASD, whose honesty contributed to chapter 7, and whose invaluable research assistance saved countless precious hours of my time. It's also richer because of the ideas, humour and constant support of Teresa Kellerman, who is an adoptive mother and FASD advocate in Tucson, Arizona; the clear observations of Donna Debolt, whose experience as a social worker in Lethbridge, Alberta, proved invaluable to me; and the many contributions of Dr. Jo Nanson, Peggy Seo Oba and Claudia Barker. Karen Palmer of the Canadian Centre for Substance Abuse and Katy Jo Fox of the University of Washington's Fetal Alcohol and Drug Unit responded promptly and patiently to my countless requests for information.

There were other generous professionals whom I consulted at various times, many of them parents of children with FASD as well: Dr. Kwadwo Asante, Mary Vandenbrink Berube, Judge Susan Carlson, Dr. Sterling Clarren, Dr. Robert Clayton, Dr. Julianne Conry, Lorian Hayes, Kay Kelly, Margaret Leslie, Diane Malbin, Chris Margetson, Kim Meawasige, Kathleen Mitchell, Allan Mountford, Barbara Neafcy, Dr. Mary D. Nettleman, Dr. Kieran O'Malley, Dr. Kathryn W. Page, Dr. Susan Rich, Dr. Christine Rogan, Dr. Robert Schacht, Barbara Smith, Dr. Brenda Stade, R.N., Dr. Ann Streissguth, the Honourable Paul Szabo, MP, Marceil Ten Eyck and Dr. Lynne Thurling.

I'm grateful for the help of Mercedes Alejandro, Gloria Armistead, Ann Gibson, Mary Horner, Jodee Kulp, Vivien Lourens, Sue Miers, Margaret Sprenger, Elspeth Ross and Shirley Winikerei, whose passionate commitment as volunteer advocates for FASD has grown out of their own family involvement. I also wish to thank the journalists Margaret Wente and Candis McLean for helping me access otherwise inaccessible media archives.

Many people from around the world trusted me enough to add their strong voices to my story: Carol Ann Allen, Corinne Barnwell, Monica Bourassa, Lori Brown, Rebecca Cave, Shona Davison, Pat De Vries, Georgianna Donnelly, Margie Fulton, Julie Gelo, Nan Gray, Cindy Haslam, Traci Henke, Johnelle Howanach and Melissa Clark, Deb Hoyt, Chris Ilomaki, Joan Kaplan, Eva Kuper, Wayne Leng, Deanna McBurney, Anne Munsch, Anne Murray, Kathryn Noxon, Judy Pakozdy, Claudia Park, Sarah Pay, Vicki Pay, Carol Peavey, Carol Ramsay, Joan Rinker, Rowena Rowley, Berna Stewart, Ryan Surbey, Angelina Taylor, Sue Truax, Fran Valentine, David Vandenbrink, Norman and Millicent Webster, Rob Wilkinson, Edith Woodward and Jennifer Woodward. I was not able to quote every one of you directly, but your experiences increased my understanding and added texture to this book.

Special thanks to Eleni Souchlas and Marie-Josee (a.k.a. MJ) Cyr for research assistance and speedy transcription of interview tapes, and to Alison Goodman of Melbourne, Australia, who knows all about writers' fragile self-esteem.

Loving gratitude to my daughter Cleo Philcox for coping with Mom's mood swings, transcribing tapes, cleaning the kitchen and, most important, giving generous permission for me to tell her part of our family's story. I'd need a whole chapter to thank Brian Philcox, my husband, partner, soulmate and editor, for his thirty-five years of love, laughter, nurturing, cheerleading and being the first reader of every chapter.

And "love always and 4ever" to Colette, for courageously encouraging me to tell her story in the hope that, as a result, fewer children will struggle lifelong with the effects of prenatal alcohol, and together all of us can begin to break the tragic cycle.

CHAPTER ONE

Rogue Sunflower

I have read that the oscillation of butterfly wings in Brazil may set off storms in Texas.
—JANETTE TURNER HOSPITAL, *THE LAST MAGICIAN*

We are all interconnected — our lives profoundly influenced by small events that may have happened years ago, involving people we may never know. Back in April of 1979, a woman addicted to alcohol, whom I have never met, became pregnant with her third child, continued to drink throughout her pregnancy — and whirled my life into an unending orbit of love, grief, despair and hope.

This woman is the reason why, one frosty December afternoon in 1997, my rusting seven-year-old white Chevy station wagon, which should be heading home to Toronto's Beaches, is drawn instead towards a seedy downtown district. At the shabby Queen-Jarvis intersection, I see five young street guys with squeegees, and slow down for a closer look. The car behind me honks. I peer at the squeegee kids as I drive past. The blond "guy" in the black toque is my eighteen-year-old daughter Colette. I drive around the block. Watching for me, she hops in with the wide, infectious grin that captured my heart when she was three.

That heart-melting grin makes me forget just how much money she has stolen from me to buy drugs, and how many lies she has told me in our years together. I don't care that she has tried every street drug going, or what she is doing with her body in order to survive. We head happily towards the nearest McDonald's. She'll have a hamburger, fries and Coke; I'm overjoyed to have fifteen minutes with my dropout homeless daughter, and listen to her tales of life on the street, sanitized for Mom.

My husband, Brian Philcox, and I have known Colette since she was ten months old. In June 1980 we had adopted our older daughter, Cleo, aged nearly three. She had been in the care of a wonderful foster family, the Newbiggings, and we had stayed in contact with them. Shortly after Cleo came to live with us, Colette was placed with the Newbiggings as a foster child. A chubby baby with big hazel eyes, a cute snub nose and a mop of curly blond hair, Colette had been taken into the care of the Children's Aid Society at age eight months because of parental neglect. Over the next two and a half years, on visits with the Newbiggings, we enjoyed Colette's spunky personality, and Cleo loved to play with her.

When Colette was nearly three, the social work agency and the courts decided that her birth parents were unable to become fit parents, and she became available for adoption. Big for her age, she had walked at eleven months, and now had a thick mane of waist-length curls. Despite numerous minor health problems in infancy—skin rashes, a mild heart murmur—she was a bright, energetic tomboy, and her foster mother worried that potential adoptive parents might be looking for a feminine child they could dress up in ruffles and ringlets. Inge, her social worker, who had been Cleo's worker as well, had a long list of applicants to choose from, and selected a couple with two school-aged sons who wanted to complete their family with a daughter.

On January 13, 1983, Colette's third birthday, Brian, Cleo and I went for a "goodbye visit," taking a present. Colette, in red overalls, was sporting an odd hairdo—one side long, one side short. When I asked what had happened to her hair, she grinned impishly, "I cutted it."

I was sunk.

When we left, she clung to us and sobbed. We hugged her goodbye, saying we'd see her soon, knowing we were lying. As we drove morosely home, Cleo, then five, broke the silence. "Why can't Colette come and live with us and be my sister?"

Brian and I explained that Cleo had always said she didn't want a sister or brother, and anyway, Inge had found a wonderful home for her. "But she could come here and I would share my room and my books and my toys," Cleo persisted.

After Cleo had gone to bed, Brian and I talked about Colette—each of us confessing we had felt a huge pang that she was going out of our lives. Who else would understand a fearless and energetic little girl who preferred trucks to dolls and was crazy about dogs and horses? Besides, she and Cleo had always played so well together. Behind Cleo's back, the discussion continued for several days.

Brian and I were both in our early forties. We had met while working in advertising in Montreal. He was unlike any other man I'd ever known—constantly cheerful, funny, a wonderful cook and an expert at ironing, sharing my interest in language, books, good food and travel and, most importantly, a guy with a huge heart. Since his early twenties, he had quietly been an international Foster Parent, supporting various families over the years. He wasn't just Mr. Right—he was my soulmate, my best friend, the person who could send me into howls of laughter at a joke nobody else would find funny, the man whose physical presence never failed to cheer and comfort me, the man I was bound to by Krazy Glue.

But could we cope with a second child? We'd been together thirteen years before our childless serenity had been shattered by Cleo's two-year-old charm, tantrums, feistiness and irresistible humour. Now, three years later, we had almost paid off the mortgage on our large old house in Toronto's beautiful Beach area. Brian was a senior executive in marketing communication, and I was a freelance journalist. We certainly weren't wealthy—but we managed to pay the bills and do lots of travelling. Could we make room in our lives and our hearts for another strong, energetic, curious little girl? Would we always kick ourselves if we didn't make the move? The answer seemed to be yes.

I took a deep breath and called Inge, the social worker. "Brian and I have been talking about this ever since Colette's birthday," I said. "If for some reason the adoption falls through—(oh, God, what am I letting myself in for?)—if this happens, we'd like to adopt Colette."

Inge reported that Colette's visit with her prospective parents had been a disaster. Taken to McDonald's, Colette had walked all over the seats and never stopped moving, much to the couple's dismay. Inge realized they were all wrong for Colette. "In fact, I've always felt she belongs with you and Brian," she said. "But you'll be getting me into big trouble. I've got twelve couples who have been approved for a little girl, and you and Brian aren't even in the pipeline."

Inge's supervisors were not happy with our attempts to "jump the queue." On Inge's suggestion, I spent a full day drafting a letter about our long-term affection for Colette, sending it to the key person in adoption at Children's Aid. She phoned me back. "That was a lovely letter, but we have many couples who have already been approved for a little girl. We can't just let you go to the head of the line." Nevertheless, she gave us an intake appointment three days later. "If the worker feels that you would be suitable parents for Colette, we will do a home study and consider you along with the other applicants. This will slow down the adoption and I'm not happy with this."

In our years in advertising, both Brian and I had put together numerous presentations, but this was the most important ever. We had forty-eight hours to convince a jaded social worker named Helen that she should make this little girl part of our family. Helped by the Newbiggings, we put together many photographs of Colette and Cleo playing together, taken at various family gatherings. When Helen asked why we felt we were the right family for Colette, we spread the pictures on her desk. Birthdays, Christmases, Easters. Cleo at three pulling ten-month-old Colette in a wagon. Two little girls hugging each other goodbye at the small family birthday a few weeks earlier.

The photos showed two children, who although unrelated biologically, bore a resemblance to each other. Race and appearance had not been important to us when we had initially applied to adopt. But, amazingly, both of these children looked exactly as our birth children might have looked. Like me, Colette was tall with thick blond hair (my grey roots now helped by the hairdresser) but, like Brian, had hazel eyes, a ski-jump nose, and a wide smile. Like me, Cleo had blue eyes and was left-handed, but her fine light brown hair was like Brian's. We hoped that Helen would view these superficial resemblances as a "good fit," though less important than the fact that we had known Colette since infancy and adored her tomboy nature.

Our strategy worked. The other twelve applicants vanished. We were thrilled to have won the battle for Colette—not realizing that this was only the first of dozens of battles we would wage on her behalf. Or with her . . .

The home study process went on for several months, and the adoption was delayed by a massive home renovation we had already put in place. We learned that despite her excellent health, Colette had a heart murmur that the doctors felt would never cause problems. We also learned that she had been removed from her birth family because of neighbours' complaints about her parents' constant drinking. Given Colette's large size and keen intelligence, the Children's Aid Society felt she had not been affected by her birth mother's addiction to alcohol.

We brought her home for good on Friday, September 22, 1980, four months before her fourth birthday, a month before Cleo turned six. Having adopted a preschooler once before, we knew the process would not be seamless, but we were not prepared for the difficulties we would have to contend with when two strong-willed little girls were brought together under one roof.

On the first Sunday after we brought Colette home, we went on a family walk to the beach, a few blocks away. It was an idyllic autumn day, warm and sunny, and the little girls played on every piece of playground equipment that lined the park and boardwalk. As we walked back up the hill home, Cleo was holding Brian's left hand. Colette grabbed his right hand, then yelled at Cleo, "You can't hold his hand! He's my dad now!"

Cleo stood in mid-sidewalk, stunned, tears in her huge blue eyes. She was sharing her room, her toys and her parents with this so-called "sister." Now this person was taking over her dad—and it had all been Cleo's own idea!

We held our first family meeting right that minute in the middle of Silverbirch Road, explaining that Brian and I both had two hands, and enough love for two little girls. But Colette had thrown down the gauntlet, and the interminable battle had begun.

It was a rocky few months. Cleo was in first grade, and Colette was spending weekday mornings in a small, excellent play group, which Cleo had also attended. In the afternoons, Colette and I would do errands and go to the park. Cleo was lost in the French immersion class she was attending. She couldn't understand French, and her teacher was not sympathetic to the stress resulting from a new sister who noisily competed for her parents' love. After several frustrating weeks, I put Cleo in a different school, English-only, and with a far more sympathetic principal and first-grade teacher.

Night after night at bedtime, Colette would sob hysterically, missing her foster parents. We all tried to comfort her, putting her into our bed, brushing her long hair, hugging her. She could not be comforted. In the series of sessions on "older-child adoption" that Brian and I had attended before adopting Cleo, we'd learned to deal with such grief by verbalizing children's feelings, and I tried this approach: "This is a hard time for you, honey. You really miss Dona and Cliff."

"It's not a hard time," she wailed. "Just take me back to Dona and Cliff and I'll be fine."

The Children's Aid Society had recommended that she not be allowed any contact with them for three months, but we allowed the odd bedtime phone call, which soothed her a little.

Despite Cleo's new, supportive teacher, she continued to struggle. Always temperamental and given to tantrums, she was mean to her sister and often a misery to live with. I do not believe in violence, and am opposed to corporal punishment. But one school morning, I could not take Cleo's ratty behaviour one more minute and was shocked to find myself dumping her bowl of Shreddies, bananas and milk over her head.

Compared to Cleo, Colette was an easy child. She and Cleo both had recurring ear infections, which meant frequent trips to our family doctor, but other than that Colette had no health problems. Cheerful, cooperative and determined, she adored animals, loved to be read to, and enjoyed building odd wooden sculptures with hammer and nails. She was fearless and stoical—climbing trees, never flinching when injured or facing a vaccination needle.

She loved practical jokes. One cold winter night, at bedtime, she vanished, and couldn't be found anywhere. Yelling desperately, the three of us searched every part of the house. Eventually, I found her, sound asleep, behind the clothes at the back of my closet. She had thought it would be a good joke to hide on us—and had fallen asleep while waiting to be found.

By the time Christmas arrived, and the entire Newbigging clan trooped in, bearing gifts and yet another foster baby, she seemed fine. Nevertheless, that first Christmas, we discovered a more disturbing facet to her personality: her uncanny ability to look us in the eye and convince us that Cleo's Christmas chocolates had magically flown out of her tin candy box. We told ourselves that Colette was not quite four, and the psychology books said that stealing was a phase. Over and over we explained the need to respect other people's property, and over and over she said she understood—and stole again.

Crazy Normalcy

But her "borrowing" seemed to be just an occasional, minor quirk. Family photos and videos show a family that looks like a cereal commercial. I look back in awe at those unruffled, energetic parents, seeming much younger than their years, enjoying the crazy normalcy. When Brian arrived home after work, I used to feel that the RCMP had arrived. The front hall had a wonderful oak staircase, and one at a time, the girls would hurl themselves at him from the landing in what they called a "jump hug."

In March 1984, Helen came to sign Colette's final adoption papers, and Brian set up the video camera on a tripod to record this historic event. We're all nicely dressed. Brian and I are sitting next to Helen on the couch, and there are tea and cookies on the coffee table. Brian and I are calmly sipping tea, rather like the Queen and Prince Philip—paying little attention to two noisy little girls who endlessly leap, spin and crash in and out of camera range, occasionally grabbing cookies and munching as they fly by. Every so often, I sweetly say things like, "Please don't scribble on the adoption papers. The judge is going to need them." (Who *is* this person?)

Colette's preschool and kindergarten teachers were enthusiastic about her gregarious nature, good verbal skills, keen interest in learning and excellent large muscle coordination. "Colette is a strong, energetic child, talkative, friendly and a joy to teach," wrote her junior kindergarten teacher in her end-of-year report:

> Each afternoon she starts out in the block centre. Here she creates all sorts of wonderful ideas from houses to camels. She initiates ideas for others to follow, and she plays cooperatively as well . . . She has an excellent vocabulary . . . She is a very social little person, sought after as a playmate by many friends. Her attention span is excellent, and she focuses well on the story line. She delights in music and loves to play musical instruments . . . She has a natural grace and sense of rhythm, and learns lyrics to new songs quickly . . . Her large muscles are well knit, and she is fearless at climbing, jumping and balancing. We will continue to encourage her fine muscle control and her hand-eye coordination.

I was too naive to understand that the line about fine muscle control and hand-eye coordination meant, "We have a real problem here." When Colette began first grade at the age of six and a half, problems erupted. By the end of first grade, when she still could not read and had great difficulty printing, I began to fight for special help for her. This was something I had already been forced to do for Cleo, who was then in third grade and had been put in a special education class half-days.

The public school the girls attended was locally famous for its nurturing atmosphere, but as we lived several kilometres away, a great deal of my time was taken up with car-pooling. Every day at 3:30, I'd wait in my car and see Colette bursting out of the school with a huge grin, free at last, her hair an unkempt mop, her parka unzipped, no mitts, no hat, in even the coldest weather. She seemed impervious to cold and pain.

Unlike Cleo, who would react to minor scrapes and scratches by shrieking to be taken to hospital, Colette rarely complained when injured. One Sunday afternoon, shortly before going to a birthday party, Colette accidentally cut her finger while peeling an apple. Brian wrapped it with gauze and tape and sent her on her way. Two hours later, the birthday child's mother phoned because the cut was still bleeding; she was a nurse, and felt that Colette should be taken to hospital for stitches. Overwhelmed with guilt, Brian took her into Emergency at our local hospital. The finger was frozen and stitched up, while Colette cheerfully looked on, so fascinated that the doctor told her that if she didn't get her nose out of the way, he'd sew it to her finger. The following day, she removed the bandage before going to school, to show off her stitches.

Her room was a disaster area: every week our cleaning woman would bring it to some degree of order and within twenty-four hours it would be a junk heap again. Brian, ex-navy and more passionate about neatness than I am, tried to get Colette to put things away on the numerous shelves that lined her large room. For years, he fought the battle and lost. I gave up early on. He also tried in vain to get her to eat one mouthful of vegetables with each meal. Parenting was an area where our own childhood experiences showed in our different approaches. Although our parents had all come of age in the Great Depression, Brian's parents had been far more strict and demanding than mine. I grew up in a relaxed, book-filled environment. My English-professor father, a gentle man with a huge heart and many talents—boxer, carpenter, cartoonist, public speaker, politician, avid golfer—was so preoccupied with his busy life that he was oblivious to what we ate or how we behaved. My mother, a former teacher, was more concerned about filling us up than whether we were getting adequate vitamins. I felt that despite Colette's hatred of broccoli, she was not suffering from malnutrition—a view that for some reason Brian could not share.

I tried different techniques for dealing with "the room." When Colette was six, I found a book that suggested involving the child in creating a bedroom that worked. Following the book's instructions, I made Colette a snack, and sat her down in the middle of the room. "Now, Colette, if there was just one change you could make to this room, what would it be?"

She thought for a moment. "I'd like it in a different house. With a different family."

At the time, I regarded this remark as just one more quirky Colette comment—not realizing it was part of an attachment problem that we would have to deal with throughout her childhood.

Much of my energy was taken up by Cleo. Shy, anxious, emotionally fragile, she was spending half-days in a highly structured special classroom for children with learning disabilities. At first, I'd been shocked by the room's bleakly bare walls and the old-fashioned firmness of Miss M., near retirement, and her elderly assistant. But Cleo flourished in that classroom and grew to love her gruff, demanding, yet kindly teacher. Unfortunately, the other half of the day was spent in a regular classroom, where she was often ignored by the teacher and bullied by some of the pupils. I complained to the principal, but despite the school's reputation as a child-centred place, nobody except Miss M. cared about a little girl whose huge blue eyes mirrored the pain she was feeling. She took out her pain by bullying the one person smaller than she was—her sister.

By the time Colette was six, she had caught up to Cleo in size. Early one Sunday morning she began to fight back. We could hear from our adjacent bedroom as Cleo began picking on her—then Cleo's shrieks of agony as Colette wrapped her fingers around a handful of her sister's fine, wavy hair and began pulling it. We thought that maybe Cleo would learn her lesson. But now, evenly matched, they fought continually and viciously, the battles spurred on by the fact that each felt that we loved the other more.

Brian travelled frequently on business, and generally brought home gifts for the girls, from places such as Nashville, New Orleans or San Francisco. He would try to find a special gift for each of them, but one always felt the other's present was better. And when he brought home identical gifts, they would be furious. Eventually he stopped bringing presents home altogether.

By second grade, Colette's reading still hadn't improved, and Cleo, in fourth grade, still had great difficulty with math. Brian and I looked on helplessly as Colette, who had been a bright, curious preschooler, lost all interest in school, becoming addicted to TV shows about animals, the bigger and scarier the better. First begging, then battling for help with both girls, I sensed that the principal and teachers dreaded my phone calls, but we needed more time than the fifteen minutes allotted on Parents' Night. To get double sessions, we bribed the teachers with coffee and Brian's home-baked chocolate chip cookies. Right to the end of elementary school, we constantly asked her teachers if there was any way we could work with Colette to help her catch up in reading, writing and math, and over and over we were told, "We're the experts. Leave the teaching to us. Just concentrate on being good parents."

Brian and I continued reading to both girls, which they loved, and tried numerous other ways of encouraging Colette to think and learn. Before she could get special help, she needed a "psychoeducational assessment," and she was placed at the end of a long waiting list. She was not tested until the end of grade three, at the age of eight and a half.

The psychologist's battery of tests indicated "overall functioning in the high average range" with superior scores "on verbal activities involving vocabulary definitions and understanding of common sense situations." She was also found to be superior in her ability to "differentiate between essential and nonessential details," and very superior "on visual performance tasks requiring non-verbal reasoning." (She demonstrated this latter ability at age eight by becoming the family expert in programming a VCR, without using a manual.) However, her decoding/reading skills were at early first grade, placing her at the 0.7 percentile—the very bottom. Spelling was at mid-grade-one level: she was only able to spell four out of eighteen simple words dictated to her. Her arithmetic was at the beginning of grade-two level. Her "visual-motor integration and fine motor control" were three years behind, and her handwriting was slow and laboured. The tester also felt that:

> Unresolved issues relating to adoption and conflict with her sister may be having an impact on her learning. She appears to tune out when not interested, therefore she has gaps in both knowledge and strategy . . . Significant intellectual strengths and weaknesses, which may be related to her difficulty were noted . . . It has been recommended to parents that they seek help to deal with emotional issues . . .

Colette was recommended for a meeting of the "Identification, Placement and Review Committee" to consider special education. I tried to find the help that had been suggested for emotional issues, but none seemed to exist. Learning support had also been recommended, but it was spotty for an entire year, though a part-time resource-room teacher did give her occasional help in reading and math. By now, having dealt with learning-disabled daughters for six years, I had become skilled at reading the coded messages in report cards. This one was written by her frustrated grade four teacher:

> Colette does participate during discussion times and is feeling more confident speaking in front of the class. Her handwork is progressing but she needs to take care with it. Colette is working on the Grade 4 Math program and it is becoming a challenge. She is unable to grasp or apply the concepts independently and requires a lot of extra time and help. Number facts are still very weak I hope she can develop stronger work habits next year to help her progress more steadily.

What this report meant was, "This kid is driving me crazy. She's way behind in math and she's careless and lazy. The one thing she can do well is talk. In fact, if she could do her schoolwork as well as she can talk in class, she'd be a much better student. She doesn't deserve to pass, but I'm going to move her to fifth grade so I don't have to cope with her again."

Colette began stealing money from us, from friends at school, and from neighbours. Whenever she was caught, I forced her to return the money and apologize, taking it out of her allowance, hoping that this humiliation would stop her—but nothing worked. Over and over we explained to her why stealing was a bad idea, imposed consequences or took away privileges. Nothing worked. She seemed to have no conscience.

By the time she was ten, I had begun to think the problem might be linked to her feelings about adoption. Brian and I tried our best in the face of her continual anger and resentment. "You're not my real parents!" and "You're not my blood!" were her two favourite expressions, often followed by a slammed door. She was angry at us for having adopted her; angry at her birth parents for having lost her. I read every psychology book I could find and kept looking for help in dealing with the adoption issue, but despite the fact that we lived in a city of three million people, resources were scanty. The Children's Aid Society, where we had adopted her, could offer no suggestions.

Every therapist and clinic had a lengthy waiting list: I called Toronto's world-renowned Hospital for Sick Children and was told there was a one-year wait list for psychiatric help. However, a few months previously, I had interviewed one of the hospital's psychiatrists for an article. I persuaded her to squeeze us in. After talking to Colette for half an hour, and administering a brief verbal test for depression, she brusquely sent me on my way with "She's a perfectly normal little girl. I'm dealing with babies with AIDS."

Our family doctor referred me to the one child psychiatrist she knew. Our first meeting with "Dr. Edwards" was not auspicious. An hour earlier, the cashier at our local supermarket had just rung up $100 worth of groceries, when I opened my wallet and found I was $40 short, although I had gone to the bank the previous day. There was only one person who could be responsible. Colette. Because the supermarket did not take credit cards, I wrote a cheque for the groceries, dropped them off at home, and drove to the school at lunchtime to pick her up for the doctor's appointment. She wasn't there. I found her at the local pizza joint, treating all of her friends—with my grocery money. Furious, I grabbed her, pulled her to the car and told her to get in. As we drove to the doctor's office, we had a huge battle, and I totally lost control. I smacked her. On the face.

I was horrified with myself. Brian and I had made a point of never hitting our children, and here I was—a child abuser! If Colette told Dr. Edwards I had hit her, or if her sensitive fair skin showed a mark, the doctor would be forced to report me to the authorities. Both children could be taken away from us. I found myself begging Colette not to mention that I'd hit her. Fortunately for both of us, avoiding the truth was never a problem for Colette. She squeezed my hand and in her usual generous way, said, "It's okay, Mom. I deserved it."

After two joint family sessions, Dr. Edwards began seeing Colette, but she was uncooperative, refusing to talk to him. He offered to see me alone to help me develop strategies to cope with Colette. My third visit was on a day when everything had gone wrong. When Dr. Edwards asked me how I was, I said truthfully, "Well, the dog ate the couch."

He didn't crack a smile. "And how do you feel about that?" he asked.

How I felt, and what I didn't say, was that humour was the one defence I had left in a situation where I was being screwed around by every professional I was dealing with. I was tired of so-called experts, none of whom could have survived twenty-four hours under the same roof with Colette. The fact that Brian and I could make each other laugh at least once a day, often making evil jokes about our children, was what kept us relatively sane, passionately in love and committed to each other and our kids. How did I feel about the dog eating the couch? Couldn't this man just laugh along with me and say, "Gee, I guess it's been a tough day."

I never went back.

We then saw a psychologist through Brian's employment assistance plan. Each session was divided into three periods. First, he would work with all four of us. Then he would talk with the girls; and then with Brian and me. After a couple of sessions, he told us that he believed the real problem was that we—Brian and I—never fought. He felt that the girls should learn that people who love each other can fight and make up, and he ordered us to have a fight during the coming week, in front of the girls. For two weeks, we just couldn't do it—fighting was not our style. On the last possible day of the third week, I reminded Brian of our assignment and told him I was going to pick a fight with him that evening.

When he came home from work, the girls noticed his new haircut. "You got your hair cut," Cleo said.

"And a pretty stupid-looking haircut, too," I said nastily. "You really look dumb."

Brian's face fell. I'd never spoken to him that way before. The girls had never heard me talk to him that way either. All three of them looked at me as if I were an axe murderer. Brian left the room, hurt—having totally forgotten our planned battle.

The next day the psychologist told us that we seemed to be pretty good parents, and what we were seeing was normal sibling rivalry. He didn't want to see us again. He had people with more serious problems, he said—his next client was a woman whose eleven-year-old son was addicted to crack. We decided to stop seeing therapists, but continued trying to figure out ways of building on Colette's wonderful strengths, particularly her love for dogs and horses.

An allergist had told us that the dark circles under Cleo's eyes and her perpetual sniffling indicated allergies, and we must not have dogs or cats. Colette, at eight, began walking neighbours' dogs. When she came home with skinned knees and bleeding hands after being dragged by a friend's huge, unmanageable mongrel, we relented. Having learned that wheaten terriers are supposedly hypoallergenic, we bought a bouncy puppy, and named him O'Grady after one of Brian's grand-mothers. (Now in her twenties, Cleo is still sneeze-free.) We also sent

Colette to an expensive riding camp two years in a row. Because both girls loved the outdoors and swimming, we joined the ranks of the cash-strapped and invested in a cabin on a pristine lake, surrounded by acres of trees and wilderness.

Trying to write screenplays, I was sidetracked by hours of dealing with the girls' schools, homework, doctors, dentists, orthodontist and the seemingly endless, budget-draining shopping for two daughters of the same size and opposing tastes, who grew out of clothing faster than you can say "Sears." But we enjoyed O'Grady, our cabin, sports, travelling, family friends, birthdays and holidays; we shared a goofy sense of humour. Viewing these videos many years later, I'm awed at the patience and affection of this couple, and wonder why the therapists blamed us for our children's problems. Despite the fact that they drove us crazy on occasion, Brian and I adored our unique, complex daughters. I thought of them as my "rogue sunflowers," those feisty flowers that sprout up magically under the bird-feeder in spring. They were valiant, beautiful, one of a kind, and unlike any other sunflowers in the world.

We worked hard at being honest and open with them, talking about adoption in a relaxed way, and answered their questions as they came up. We celebrated the anniversaries of their adoption, along with birthdays. We told them that if they wanted to meet their birth parents when they were older, that was okay with us. They'd *always* be our daughters, but they had a right to know these people and have a relationship with them if they chose. I still believe that you can't have too many people who love you.

Sex was another area of frequent discussion. As a little girl, I had been sexually harassed by a male adult in my family. In adulthood, I discovered that he had also harassed my sister and female cousins. I had been afraid to tell my parents, who always quickly closed down any conversation relating to sex. I was determined that this was not going to happen to my daughters.

Unlike slim, boyish Cleo, Colette had a curvy body that began to mature by the time she was eight, something she camouflaged by wearing baggy, loose clothes. At ten and a half, Colette told me, terrified, that she must have injured herself when climbing a tree earlier that day: she was bleeding from the vagina, and it wouldn't stop. My lengthy hours of discussion about menstruation with both girls hadn't "taken." Trying to hide my sinking heart, I gave her a hug and welcomed her to the world of womanhood. Interested only in riding horses and playing with dogs, Colette reminded me of something the movie star Elizabeth Taylor (another animal lover) said about herself in early puberty: "I was a child in a woman's body."

She had been the biggest in her class since kindergarten, and by sixth grade Colette was taller than most of her teachers—five foot six, with feminine curves on her sturdy frame. But she was awkward, her former grace diminished by a maturing body she wasn't accustomed to. The year Colette was eleven and a half we went on a spring-break trip to Jamaica, where we stayed in a condo with a broken TV set. Bored, Colette picked up one of Cleo's juvenile mystery books. Two weeks in the sun accomplished what three years of special education had failed to do: she "clicked" with reading and raced through several of her sister's books. Meanwhile, her thick, curly, honey-blond hair and stunning body wowed the local young studs, who were hitting on her at every opportunity—something she was too innocent to realize.

She now slouched perpetually, attempting to look shorter and hide her breasts. School photos show a sullen adolescent with lank, greasy hair and a sprinkling of pimples. Our attempts at any kind of relationship with her were often met with rebellion, and the "social little person" of kindergarten now had few friends except three tough young boys with similar learning problems and a neighbour girl, three years younger, who shared her passion for animals. But she hadn't lost her great physical strength. At one interschool softball game I attended she slouched to the plate and hit three grand-slam home runs. Even her attempts at cool couldn't mask the small smile of pride each time she loped across home plate. On her final, game-winning run, as her schoolmates and their parents leapt to their feet and cheered, I found myself weeping.

She graduated from sixth grade a few weeks later, wearing her favourite and only skirt: blue denim, now very short and tight, topped with a new white blouse. Our hairdresser had pulled her long hair into an elegant French braid. Shyly beautiful, six months from her thirteenth birthday, she could have passed for twenty.

CHAPTER TWO

Demon Angel

Death is a raincoat to all my problems.
Death is a Dovay [duvet] which dosent do a godd job at
    Keeping you warm.
Death is a holiday in which you all ways have no end.
Death is Forebibbin in my Mom's mind.
Death is the way to get away From all my Problems.

Rain is Falling on my head. like alot of other things as well.
                    —Poem by Colette, January 1996

Brian and I could barely remember what it felt like to be financially secure. In 1990, concerned that Cleo, shy, sensitive and learning-disabled, would sink in our neighbourhood's large "senior public school" (junior high), we'd sent her to private school. For two years a whopping chunk of his salary vanished each month, as the school cashed a series of postdated cheques. Consumed with my daughters' problems, I now made little income from writing. We had looked forward to Cleo's return to public school after eighth grade, viewing it as a return to financial stability.

But as Cleo approached graduation, we realized that if Colette were given the freedom of public junior high, she was likely to become a seventh grade dropout. Remortgaging our house, we sent Colette to the same private school, where she was placed in a highly structured special education classroom with seven other off-the-wall kids. The special ed teacher, "Mr. Connolly," a Kevin Kline look-alike, was a superhip combination of standup comic and prison guard. The walls were decorated with blow-ups of each student, looking cool in Mr. Connolly's black leather jacket. Charismatic, creative, witty, demanding, Mr. Connolly reached Colette as no previous teacher had, pushing her academically for the first time in her life. He forced her to write a journal. When her work was not completed, he made her stay after school. Grudgingly, she learned to spell and do math.

> As Colette has gained confidence, her expressive language style has become more appropriate and communicative. She has changed dramatically in her attitude and this is evident in the way she uses her voice and her willingness to express different viewpoints. There are significantly fewer "one syllable" responses to questions asked of her. Colette's attentiveness has improved considerably this year. . . . (School Report, June 1993)

To save money, we cancelled our expensive Y membership and joined Variety Village, a fitness and rehabilitation centre offering special facilities—and discounts—for disabled people. For once, our daughters' learning disabilities gave us a financial benefit. To our surprise, Colette, now thirteen, decided to join the Village swim team, coached by the marathon swimmer Vicki Keith, who had swum all five Great Lakes. Joining the team of young disabled and non-disabled swimmers, kids with infectious energy and humour, Colette became highly motivated for the first time in her life. She had remarkable strength and endurance, and the longer the swim, the better she did. We took turns driving her to swim meets, and Brian took classes to become a swim meet official, car-pooling young swimmers all over Southern Ontario.

In the summer of 1993 Colette's swimming buddy and mentor, Carlos Costa, tackled the twenty-six-mile swim across frigid Lake

Ontario. Handsome, determined, bright and funny, twenty-year-old Carlos had been born with deformed legs that had been amputated when he was two years old. Colette, Brian, the swim team and busloads of disabled children cheered him on for hours, baking in the August sun at the water's edge as he fought freezing currents and ten-foot waves. He was the first physically challenged swimmer to conquer one of the Great Lakes—and Colette was thrilled and inspired. Later that fall, she came to Brian and me, and said in a shy, offhand way, "I've been thinkin' . . . If I swam the lake next summer, I'd be the youngest person ever. I'd be fourteen. I'd be younger than Marilyn Bell or Cindy Nicholas." (Bell and Nicholas were famous teenaged Canadian marathon swimmers.) What d'you guys think?"

Stunned but delighted, we told her that we'd do our best to help: drive her to early-morning training sessions, find corporate sponsors, get a boat and support team in place. A few days later, Vicki Keith approached me near the pool, and asked if Colette had mentioned her idea for swimming Lake Ontario. "I think she can do it," Vicki said. "She's got the right body; she's strong and determined. If she wants to do it, I'll work with her."

By now we had acquired a second wheaten terrier, Misty, a cuddly flaxen blond doggie Marilyn Monroe, and had mated her with raffish Jiggs, owned by my friend Keitha McLean. In September 1993 Misty gave birth to eight wheaten puppies, assisted by midwife Colette. While I, flustered, flipped the pages of library books about breeding puppies, reading appropriate passages aloud, Colette calmly caught the puppies as they emerged, snipped the umbilical cords, opened the sacs, dried the pups and placed them on a heating pad. At age seven, she had been thrilled to assist in the delivery of a calf on a dairy farm. Now, at thirteen, she was in her element—tender, loving, unsqueamish. To Cleo the whole process was yucky; she couldn't bear to look. As for Brian, he was conveniently away on a business trip.

Brian had built a giant whelping box/nursery, which took over our breakfast room, and Colette stayed up for the puppies' first three nights, making sure all were fed and warm. We named the first and toughest

"Vicki," after Vicki Keith, and a small, feisty male became "Carlos" after Colette's hero, the lake swimmer. Misty was not a natural mother, but because of Colette's excellent care, seven of the eight puppies survived. At thirteen, she did not know her times tables and still reversed many letters, but I was awed by her gift at working with animals.

Colette seemed to have her life on track, but Cleo was on a downward slide. That summer, she had gone on a student exchange to Quebec and instead of learning French had come home with her first boyfriend. "Kevin" was clever, athletic, gentle, supportive and as enamoured of Cleo as she was of him. All fall she had been walking on air, but as winter approached she became increasingly unhappy. Brian, Kevin and I were puzzled: what was wrong with her? Weepy, miserable and impossible to live with, she couldn't articulate what the problem was. Even her Christmas presents failed to comfort her. When we adopted Cleo, we'd been informed that both birth parents had struggled with depression: could she have inherited this problem? Early in the New Year, I began my search for a psychiatrist.

The doctor diagnosed severe depression and began trying a series of antidepressants, each of which made her more zombie-like than the previous one. It became impossible to get her out of bed, and her school year was in jeopardy. I seemed to be spending most of my time driving around in snowstorms with Cleo and waiting outside the psychiatrist's office.

Meanwhile, Colette had volunteered to officiate at wheelchair basketball games. Unfortunately, in a gymnasium full of keen wheelchair athletes, she zeroed in on a small group of people who blunted the pain of their disabilities with drugs. The weekend of Brian's and my twenty-third wedding anniversary, in February 1994, she stayed over at the home of "Susie," a young woman with cerebral palsy. They planned to attend a birthday party for "George," a quadriplegic young adult man who lived in a residence for disabled people.

She didn't return until late Sunday afternoon. Alarm bells went off for me. The next day, Cleo, worried, told us what Colette had told her: that there was lots of marijuana at the party, and that she'd had sexual relations with one of the men, a twenty-four-year-old dealer. I confronted Colette—who was furious with her sister for squealing—and took her to our family doctor. I called the residence for disabled people: they didn't care that the party had involved drugs and sexual activities with minors. I also called the police, and was told that in Canada, fourteen is the age of sexual consent: unless Colette pressed charges, there was nothing we could do. The police seemed equally unconcerned that a fourteen-year-old girl had been given marijuana and encouraged to have sex with a stranger ten years her senior.

Everything was falling apart. Cleo's depression was not getting better, and Colette had quit swimming. Not only that, Colette was smoking cigarettes regularly and using God-knows-what other drugs. Copying a favourite rock star, she had shaved her head at the back and sides, dyed the remainder black and pulled it back in a ponytail. ("Y'look like you got a dead squirrel on your head," said her friend Susie.) Returning from school each day, wearing her tartan school kilt and high-top Doc Marten boots, she would stomp upstairs without saying hello. Then heavy metal music would blast from her room, while she lay on her bed. Her room, always a disaster, now looked as if it had been struck by a Florida hurricane. Using a black felt-tip marker, she'd written the lyrics of heavy metal music on the walls, adding illustrations of devils and knives dripping with blood.

Thursday Nights in a Circle

I'd like to remind you of the code of confidentiality. Everything said in the group, remains in the group. Are there any announcements? Any court dates?

—OPENING WORDS, PARENT SUPPORT GROUP

A support group for parents of acting-out teenagers met on Thursday nights at Cleo's high school, and I began attending. For the first time, I was among people who were familiar with the same frustration and despair I had experienced. We all seemed to have the same demon child, who lied, stole, used drugs, was sexually promiscuous, refused to attend school—a child who nevertheless could sometimes be sweet and loving. A box of tissues sat in the middle of the floor for the inevitable tears of newcomers, and when I told my story for the first time, I used a lot of them.

The small neighbourhood group is part of a province-wide charitable organization called Association of Parent Support Groups in Ontario (APSGO), which, organizers were careful to point out, is nothing like the "Tough Love" movement. At the first meeting, I was asked to make a list of all of the stuff Colette did that drove me crazy, and then divide it into two piles: the things that were her problem, and the things that were my problem. I was also asked to purchase a book called *How to Deal with Your Acting-Out Teenager.*

Authors Bayard and Bayard said that school attendance, homework, sexual activities, appearance and use of alcohol and drugs were part of your child's pile and generally should be ignored. My pile included her ear-splitting rock music, swearing, physical abuse, theft, vandalism—and those were things I could work on eliminating. (Oh, yeah? Hadn't I already tried to do so?) The authors told parents to stop yelling, screaming, preaching, grounding, punishing, trying to control. Instead, we were advised to set clear personal boundaries, figure out ways of ensuring that our child must take responsibility for his or her actions—involving the police if necessary—ask few questions, keep our lips zipped, leave the room or even the house instead of fighting. Most important, we were to work at building a good relationship with him or her. It sounded crazy, but what did I have to lose?

Representing many ethnic groups and ranging from welfare mothers to professionals, the other parents—mostly women—were as bewildered as I was. We loved our children and were doing the best we could, but were being blamed by schools, the police, courts and therapists. I began to take the group's free workshops, and within six months found myself running meetings, eventually winding up on both the provincial board and the executive. Many parents quickly learned the techniques, built better relationships with their children and "graduated"—but for me those Thursday nights in a circle lasted for nearly six years. A handful of those women held my hand on that long, rocky roller-coaster ride, and to them, I will be eternally grateful.

Easter Monday, 1994. Brian had left on a business trip to Philadelphia. I snuggled into bed at nine o'clock with a paperback thriller and a grilled cheese sandwich—then heard a ruckus from the kitchen. Throwing on my robe, I ran downstairs to find Cleo talking on the phone to her boyfriend Kevin, while Colette held a giant bread knife to her sister's throat, screaming, "I'm gonna kill you!"

It seems that Cleo had eaten the end of Colette's chocolate Easter bunny—a thumb-size morsel she had left near the front hall telephone. The previous week, I had come in the door to find the girls fighting in the upstairs hall, Cleo prostrate on the floor shrieking, while Colette kicked her with her Doc Marten boots. She would not stop until I picked up the phone and began dialing 911. Cleo still had bruises.

Heart pounding, I told Colette to put down the knife.

"You can't make me."

"I'll call the police," I said.

"You don't have the guts."

"Oh, yeah?" I went to the hall phone.

The trouble was, I couldn't call the police, because Cleo was talking on our only line, in the kitchen . . . with a knife to her throat. "She's threatening me with a knife," she said calmly to Kevin. "Stop it, Colette, go away." In retrospect, ignoring her sister and continuing to talk on the phone normally was a good method of cooling down a potentially explosive situation.

By now it was 10:00 p.m., and I found myself in my robe and slippers, pounding on my neighbours' door. I woke them up and used their phone to call the police.

When I got back, Colette was innocently leafing through a *National Geographic* and Cleo was still on the phone.

There were sirens. Two women police officers came in, and Cleo and I independently told our stories. By this time, Cleo was in shock, shaking and crying. The police asked if we wanted to press charges, and both of us had had enough. We said, "Yes."

When they took Colette away, I thought they'd merely scare her a little. Instead, they locked her up overnight, and one of the female officers arrived back around 1:00 a.m., with a "Notice to Parents" advising me of a bail hearing the following morning.

"She wasn't like other kids we see," the officer said. "She was polite and respectful. Please be there for her tomorrow. She needs you." My early night turned into a wide-awake nightmare, compounded by the fact that Brian was not answering the phone in his Philadelphia hotel room. I left numerous urgent messages asking him to call home. When he still wasn't answering at six the next morning, I felt sure our marriage was over.

The next morning I watched, exhausted and hollow-eyed, as Colette was brought into the courtroom in handcuffs, terrified. And I was the one who had put her there. They put her in the prisoners' box with a couple of tough-looking boys. She looked out into the courtroom, and our eyes met. Trying to look encouraging, I nearly lost it when the crown attorney asked her, "Do you have a lawyer?" She looked at me again, and said, in the voice of a frightened four-year-old, "I don't know. You'll have to ask my mom."

She was charged with assault with a deadly weapon and uttering death threats, and remanded until after lunch. I checked my voice-mail and found an anxious message from Brian. The hotel management had moved him to a different room, and the operator didn't know and had been ringing me through to the wrong room all night. Relieved that he still loved me, I left yet another message at the right room, blurting out the whole story. Then I hunted down the duty lawyer, who brusquely told me the judge would not allow Colette to go home with me, as she would be viewed as a threat to her sister's safety. Somewhere in that courthouse, I managed to find a really good lawyer who put me on the stand that afternoon. I told the judge about life with Colette, and convinced him that if she did anything like that again, I would pull the bail.

While waiting to sign the $500 bond, I went to the washroom to do something about my unkempt appearance. A fiftyish woman approached me. "I heard you in the courtroom," she said. "Your story is so much like mine. My daughter is adopted too, and I've been going to APSGO (the parent support group) for years. I just wanted to wish you good luck."

After I signed, I was allowed to take Colette home, on condition that she go to school, attend drug and alcohol rehab, agree to counselling, be home by 7:00 p.m. every evening and rejoin the swim team. As we drove home, she launched into a tirade. The previous night, they had taken away her Doc Martens boots and made her wear baby blue sneakers with Velcro tabs. "Since when is saying I'M GONNA KILL YOU a death threat?"

For the next few months, she fulfilled all her bail conditions. She was back on the swim team and staying away from her druggie wheelchair friends. In all Ontario I could not find a residential rehab facility that would accept a fourteen-year-old female, but Brian drove her to regular Narcotics Anonymous meetings, which she seemed to enjoy. As the court suggested, we saw yet another counsellor. This social worker, herself a young mother with two children, felt that our negativity had been the root cause of our problems with Colette, and asked us to return each week with a list of the positive things that Colette had done. Once again, I wondered how long this counsellor would have survived the stress that Brian and I had endured for so many years.

Having had the good luck to grow up with loving parents, and having found a supportive life partner, I had always considered myself a strong and happy person who didn't need psychiatric help. But because of my children's problems, I'd spent the greater part of the past few years sitting with them in the offices of various professionals. Now, in order to keep going, I was attending weekly group therapy, given by a psychiatrist and psychologist.

When the case finally went to court in late June, Colette was neat and beautiful in a blazer, white shirt and school kilt, her hair in a blond pageboy artfully combed so that the shaved spots didn't show. Her lawyer spoke eloquently about how she had rebuilt her life. Pleading guilty, she told the judge she was really, really sorry and had learned her lesson. Bamboozled by her tears and angelic charm, the judge, to my horror, gave her an absolute discharge. No probation. No curfew. No rules.

She was never violent with her sister again, and managed to complete her school year, but within a few days of her graduation from eighth grade a new problem appeared. She was vanishing for days on end. The three of us could be watching TV, she'd go upstairs to fix something to eat—and be gone. After a few days, we'd again report her as missing, and when she resurfaced, we'd report that she was no longer missing. Each time we filed one of these reports, a police officer would arrive at the door. The officers advised us that they would not search for her, and as she was fourteen, they could not force her to come home. However, they recommended that we file a missing persons report each time she vanished, in case she was found injured or dead. The neighbours became used to the police car in front of our house.

Most of our friends felt we were insane to put up with Colette's behaviour, but my close friend of thirty years, Keitha McLean, a brilliant writer and editor, encouraged us to keep going. Back in the seventies, Keitha had become cross-addicted to alcohol and Valium, and we had supported her during her rehabilitation. Sober since 1976, Keitha had become an expert on addiction, and now edited a fascinating magazine called *Pathways,* devoted to recovery issues. She had always related to Colette's tomboy strengths, and having witnessed so many AA miracles, believed that at some point Colette too would find herself.

One day, Keitha said, "Did it ever occur to you that Colette might have fetal alcohol syndrome?" I pointed out that as far as I knew, people with FAS were small and severely mentally disabled. The Children's Aid doctors had felt that Colette's birth mother's drinking hadn't affected her, and although I had mentioned her birth parents' alcoholism to every psychiatrist and therapist we had seen, nobody had suggested FAS. "Well, it might be fetal alcohol effects, " said Keitha.

"Maybe you should look into it." It seemed unlikely, and I put it out of my mind.

Instead, I tried to figure out what was motivating Colette. Adoption continued to be a major issue with her, and Brian and I felt it might be helpful if she met her half-brother "Freddie," the son of her birth mother, five years older than she. Freddie had been in a foster home with a caring single mother who could not afford to adopt him, but wanted to keep him permanently. Unfortunately, as he hit his teens, this loving woman died, and he had spent his adolescence in a series of foster homes. Freddie and Colette had not seen each other since Colette was a toddler, but her "big brother" had assumed mythic, white-knight proportions in her mind.

The Children's Aid Society found Freddie for Colette. That summer, 1994, Colette talked to him on the phone, and Brian made the three-hour drive with her to the city where he was living on welfare. Long and lanky, Freddie had Colette's colouring and laconic personality; she was entranced by her big brother. Freddie enjoyed meeting her, but did not share her enthusiasm for building a relationship. Eventually he vanished, and she has never heard from him again. We tried to explain to her that his life had been so difficult that he was unable to love and trust anyone, even her—not an easy concept for a troubled fourteen-year-old to understand. (We now believe that Freddie has been repeatedly in and out of jail.)

COLETTE'S WILL

To whom it may concern! If I may die I wish to be berried
and the heading on the tombstone should read like this
"SHE LIVED A METALERS LIFE STYLE! AND WAS CRAZY FOR MARIJUANA!"

I am giving almost all of my SHIT (stuff) to my family
and if they don't want it then they can give it to good will.
I'm giving my boyfriend dizzy my necklace with the raven and the dove

pendants on it, the ring on my left hand on the fourth finger,
and the dried rose hanging from the bulletin bored in my room.

AND TO THE REST WHO I LEFT OUT
LOVE YOU FOREVER AND ALWAYS
COLETTE

This will was written in September 1994, and found five years later on a computer disk in my office. If Brian and I had discovered it earlier, we would have been even more terrified for Colette's safety. Over the summer of 1994, the drug use, rages and disappearances continued, and I begged the Children's Aid Society for respite—a foster home or group home—but they refused to help. The youth worker told us that, as Colette was adopted, she was our responsibility and there was nothing they could do. I told the psychiatrist and psychologist at my weekly group therapy session what I was going through.

"Every week you come here and you tell us about how awful your daughter is," said the male psychologist. "If I told you I wanted to lose weight, but every week I came back fat, what would you think?"

"I'd think you didn't really want to lose weight," I said.

"Exactly," he said triumphantly. "Have you put her and her clothes on the porch and told Children's Aid they have to come and take her?"

I told him that she was stronger than I was. Besides, any physical conflict could escalate into injury, a visit from the police and criminal charges. As well, throwing her out would be illegal and probably result in our being charged with abandonment. Finally, despite her terrible behaviour and exterior bravado, I knew that inside she was lonely and vulnerable, and needed us. The psychologist threw up his hands. "When my son was sixteen, I threw him out and never let him come back," he said. "Best thing for both of us." I quit the group and instead spent the summer on the phone, burning up the phone lines in search of a miracle.

In September, that miracle appeared in the form of the C. M. Hincks Children's Mental Health Centre. I had phoned them earlier that summer and been told there was a seven-month wait for an intake appointment. They had sent me a lengthy application form, which I had filled out and returned, along with a three-page letter about our fears for Colette's safety. Amazingly, they'd had a cancellation and could fit us in for an intake appointment the following week, only two months after I had applied. Getting her there was the only problem. She was skipping school, and it was only a matter of time until she vanished again. We took her out of school and spent the rest of the week at our isolated cabin, then made the three-hour drive directly from there to the Hincks clinic.

The intake interviewer talked with the four of us while two psychiatrists behind a one-way glass window looked on. Colette displayed her usual anger and bravado. Brian, Cleo and I spoke emotionally about our great pain at her behaviour, and our fears for her life. "I don't give a fuck," Colette said. "I don't care whether I live or die."

In fact, she did care. She had received two terrifying phone calls—death threats from men she'd met on the street. She was furious at us for not reporting them to the police. But there were no witnesses; it would have been her word against theirs.

We managed to get her in for the follow-up appointment the next week. The intake worker was the first of all of the therapists we had consulted who did not blame us for Colette's behaviour. "You have a real problem," she told Brian and me. "We don't know how you've managed to survive so well for so long."

Then she turned to Colette. "Sometimes when people seem angry, they're really afraid," she told her. "Your mom and dad are afraid for your life, and we're afraid too."

"Well, I'm not afraid—" Colette began to bluster, but the worker cut her off.

"We have a place where teenagers can be safe. It's a farm, up north."

"Does it have horses?"

"No, but it has cows and pigs and sheep and turkeys and chickens."

Thinking that it would be nice to get out of town for a few weeks until her street problems died down, animal-loving Colette jumped at the chance. Two weeks later, I took her to sign documents for her voluntary committal. The worker asked her to read the papers carefully, and as she scanned them, I held my breath. Afraid for her safety in the city, she hadn't asked me how long she would be at Hincks. I'd always made a point of not lying to my children, ever—but in this instance, I hadn't volunteered the information. Her learning disabilities may have saved her life: she signed, not realizing she had just committed herself to a two-year residential treatment program.

> Colette has difficulty exploring the reasons for her problems and acting out, wanting to minimize past serious incidents. She is quite defended [has put up many defences] about whatever guilt and remorse she may feel for the turmoil that has occurred in the family and tends to externalize blame. She has tested out constantly her parents' commitment to her over the years, which is commonly the case with kids who are adopted later. . . . She would much prefer not to discuss issues that are painful to her and has trouble tolerating her sadness. She will try to distract and derail the conversation from such areas, using temper outbursts, tears and threats to avoid. (Psychiatrist's notes, C. M. Hincks Rural Treatment Centre, November 25, 1994)

On October 25, 1994, we drove Colette up to the C. M. Hincks Rural Treatment Centre, a.k.a. "the Farm," about two hours north of Toronto. The idyllic Farm is set amid apple orchards and horse stables, high above a scenic valley near Lake Huron's Georgian Bay. But Colette saw none of this. What she saw was her freedom vanishing. Brian took a photo of the two of us, Colette with punk hairdo and nose ring, looking bleak and terrified, me hugging her, beaming with relief.

The Farm wasn't what you might expect. It didn't look anything like a psychiatric treatment centre: there wasn't a white coat or speck of hospital-green paint in sight. The main building was rather like a large farmhouse, and there were several barns and outbuildings, a laundry, a washroom facility with showers, sinks and toilets—males on one side, females on the other—and several small, rustic cabins about a hundred feet from the washrooms. The seventeen teenagers, six of them girls, lived two to a cabin and were encouraged to decorate these spaces as they chose. A relative state of neatness was required. Going to the bathroom, even in midwinter, necessitated a hike to the washroom facility. Everybody had to participate in grocery shopping, cooking, cleaning and farm chores.

Between the time of her arrival and the assessment meeting a month later, we had numerous phone calls from Colette and talked with staff many times. She was cheerful and cooperative, they reported. She pitched in with domestic and farm chores, and was a pleasure to have around. We began to worry that they might think she didn't need to be there.

But the assessment-review meeting on November 24 ended that fear. Cleo's boyfriend, Kevin, had broken up with her, and she was so depressed that we were afraid to leave her alone. We took Cleo and both dogs to the meeting, and Colette threw one of her temper tantrums when we said she could not come home that weekend for a visit. She swore, yelled, cried and finally grabbed the dogs and stalked from the room, slamming the door. The psychiatrist (whom I'll call "Dr. McGinley"), a feisty Irish grandmother, asked us with a quizzical smile, "How do you keep from decking her?"

Unlike any of the other professionals we had consulted, the Hincks staff were realistic about the demands of coping with out-of-control teenagers twenty-four hours a day, and were aware of the enormous stress that their parents were usually under. Despite Colette's great gains during her two years in private school, she was still far behind. The Hincks tests indicated that, at the beginning of grade nine, she was two years behind in paragraph understanding, at fifth-grade level in spelling and word discrimination, and at fourth-grade level in math. In a self-administered profile called the Achenbach test, she had scored 19 out of 22 on Delinquent Behaviour and 21 out of 38 on Aggressive Behaviour, putting her well above the norm for a female of her age.

Many times during the next two years, I found myself wishing that the Hincks program could last forever for Colette. The live-in counsellors were young, energetic and committed to the kids. Every minute of the day was structured with school, chores, farm activities and recreation. Treatment consisted of informal one-on-one counselling, given while both staff member and teenager mucked out a barn or washed dishes, frequent group discussions and courses in specific areas. One course, in anger management, taught Colette how to control her rages and tantrums using the same simple techniques—take deep breaths, keep your mouth shut, get out of the environment that's making you angry—that I learned in my support group. She still uses them routinely.

It occurred to me that the Hincks approach, with its structure, rules and supervision, was the exact opposite of the laid-back philosophy recommended by my support organization. Nevertheless, I continued to attend my local group, coordinated meetings and served on the provincial board and executive. I liked the members, enjoyed their humour, warmth and support, and was glad to help newcomer parents who, like me, had been told by professionals for years that they were the cause of their children's terrible behaviour.

The Hincks counsellers knew from sad experience that success with these children did not come easily. What worked in theory did not always work in real life. One Colette quirk that did not improve under the Hincks regime was her inability to learn from a reward-consequences system. There were three levels of privileges. Every teenager came in at Level 1, and with good behaviour could earn his or her way up to more privileges in Level 2. With more good behaviour, he or she would reach the coveted Level 3, resulting in even more privileges.

The team decided that Colette's desire to work as a volunteer at a horse farm was a Level 3 privilege, and by summer she had earned her way up to that level. She loved working with the giant Hanoverian hunter horses at the nearby stable, mucking out stalls and grooming the horses. The problem was, she kept shooting herself in the foot and getting "busted" back to Level 1.

The Farm had been declared a smoke-free zone, but by Colette's second year she was attending a nearby high school, and there was nothing we could do to prevent her smoking there. We finally told

Hincks management that, although we were not happy about her smoking at school, this would have to be her decision. But the other Hincks parents had said their children were not allowed to smoke. Every time Colette reached Level 3, her friend "Tina" from the Hincks would request a cigarette outside the school, and Colette would give it to her. The other Hincks kids would report both of them, and Tina and Colette would be busted down a level. A few days later, Tina would ask for a cigarette again, and again their Hincks friends would report them, and they would be demoted to Level 1. Colette would be devastated at the loss of privileges, but could never grasp that, in order to stay at Level 3 and work with horses, she must not give Tina a cigarette. (Two years later, Brian and I would learn that her problem in understanding consequences was among her learning disabilities.)

During her nineteen months at the Farm, she complained a lot, but was safe and drug-free, completed grades nine and ten, and was well behaved on her frequent weekends at home. But the rest of our lives were in turmoil. In late 1994, while we were attending a play, Brian suddenly became deaf in one ear, and had to learn to live with perpetual tinnitus. Around the same time, Cleo was diagnosed with seasonal affective disorder (SAD), chronic depression that becomes worse in winter—something possibly inherited from her birth family. We were glad to have a name for the sadness and lethargy that attacks her every winter, and the SAD is now under control, thanks to medication and Cleo's determination.

In January 1995 my mother, who had been suffering from dementia, died suddenly in her seniors' residence in Vancouver, aged eighty-six. In February, when my close friend Keitha's Jeep slid off an icy highway, she miraculously escaped death, only to be diagnosed with terminal cancer on May 1. I painted over the devils and demons in Colette's mostly unused room and invited my long-time friend to live there for whatever time remained to her—and when Colette heard about it she was so infuriated that she threw one of her tantrums at a Hincks review session. She shouted and stormed, I wept, and Dr. McGinley lost her professional cool. "Do you ever think of anyone but yourself?" she asked Colette, while Brian and I looked on, amazed.

To her credit, Colette put her anger management techniques to good use. She excused herself and returned twenty minutes later, eyes red and teary. "I'm sorry, Mom," she said, hugging me. "I don't know what got into me. It's okay. She can use my room." I hugged her back, thanking her for her generosity.

A few weeks later, the girls' former foster mother, Dona, died suddenly of cancer, and Colette lost a source of unconditional love and support. At her graveside on that hot day in June, Dona's three children, two grandchildren and Colette each placed a red rose on her casket—Colette's rose for herself but also symbolic of those thirty-five foster children Dona had nurtured and loved enough to let go, and of whom only our daughters had continued to have contact with this warm and caring woman.

Keitha did not use Colette's room for long. She died in hospital in August, surrounded by her family, when we were at our cabin. Colette was with me when I received the news, hugging me, telling me she loved me. In the first eight months of 1995 I had lost two of the key people in my life and Colette had lost her first real mother. As well, downsizing had affected Brian's work in the large corporation where he had worked for eighteen years as a senior executive. His workload increased in volume, and the staff members that remained to him were also overworked, and feared for their jobs. He realized that what was happening to his department was part of a worldwide trend, but that didn't make it any easier.

I dreaded Colette's "graduation" from the Farm in June 1996. There was no way we could provide the structure and support of the Hincks or that country setting hundreds of miles from the drug scene. Nevertheless, we enjoyed a brief, delightful, honeymoon. That summer, near our country cabin, she rescued a huge, injured hound who had probably been mauled by a bear. Naming him Harold, she nursed him back to health, and until we found an adoptive home for him two years later, we had a three-dog household.

She stopped fighting with her sister, and hung around with Brian, playing pool and building a doghouse for Harold. The four of us had our best Christmas in years, with Colette cheerful and cooperative and Cleo's annual depression under control.

Colette was attending a transition classroom operated by the Hincks in a regular high school: half-days in a regular classroom, half-days in a special education class. For the first six months of the school year she attended school regularly and got good grades, but then in February 1997, as I washed dishes at the kitchen window, I happened to see her buying drugs from the neighbourhood youth I knew to be a dealer. In retrospect, I should probably have confronted her on the spot. Instead, I kept quiet, and raised my concerns at the next support group meeting. My friends there assured me that this was merely a "blip"—but I knew in my gut that we were facing another round of stealing and addiction, and I was right.

Brian was offered a retirement package, and, relieved at getting out of his stressful workplace, he jumped at the opportunity, retiring on March 1, 1997. But he was also secretly terrified: just as we were digging ourselves out of the financial hole we'd gotten into because of the girls' private schooling, we faced a huge drop in income. What was he going to do with his life, and how were we going to survive financially? As a twenty-sixth anniversary gift, I offered to buy him office furniture. He chose the most reasonably priced he could find, took over the basement TV room and began to explore options.

We worked hard at maintaining a good relationship with Colette, but all we could do was look on helplessly as she began to stay out past the curfew we'd all agreed on, then many nights didn't come home at all. Her two years at the Hincks and lengthy work with the Farm's counsellors had managed to keep her safe and out of trouble, but had not eliminated her inner demons. We were back at square one, only this time she was seventeen and so close to being an official adult that there was nothing we could do.

One day in March 1997 I bleakly switched on the TV set and learned that CBC-TV's public affairs show, *The National*, was going to feature a segment on fetal alcohol effects (FAE). Wasn't that what Keitha had mentioned many years earlier? I made sure to watch the program, which featured two young Vancouver men, both adopted, who had been recently diagnosed with FAE—brain damage caused by their birth mothers' drinking in pregnancy. In speech, demeanour and behaviour, Jean-François Lepage and Mark Steeves were exactly like Colette. Normal in appearance and intelligence, they actually had highly impulsive and addictive personalities; they lied, stole, had been involved with the law and seemed to have no remorse or conscience. They too had family histories that included alcoholic birth mothers and caring, bewildered, middle-class adoptive families. As vulnerable as Colette, they could also be loveable and a joy to have around: attractive, charming, funny and gifted with animals.

I was stunned. Seven minutes on television had given me what seven years of psychologists, psychiatrists, social workers and counsellors had failed to deliver: the key to the mysteries of Colette's unfathomable brain.

CHAPTER THREE

Crashing into the Iceberg

It appeared to us . . . that fetal alcohol syndrome as we know it is just the tip of the iceberg. It's visible above the surface because of the face and the physical features that are associated with it but there's a lot more below the waterline that you can't see . . . the danger lurks beneath the surface. What you see in an iceberg is like a warning. It says to you "Hey! There's a lot more below the surface that you can't see and that could cause you a ton of trouble."

—Ann Streissguth, Ph.D.

My God, Gray, the Titanic *has struck a berg!*

—Jack Goodwin, wireless operator at Cape
Race, Newfoundland, April 14, 1912

Flash forward eight months to November 1997. Colette, not yet eighteen, is addicted to crack and living on the street. She is one of the legions of tough young people with squeegee mops and pails, stopping downtown Toronto motorists and asking to clean their windshields. Desperate, fearing for her life, Brian and I are sitting in a packed auditorium in a community college in Ann Arbor, Michigan, listening to a tiny, vivacious woman with a huge smile, sparkling blue eyes, an

Einstein-like halo of curly white hair, and beneath it, a brain like Einstein's as well. She is Ann Streissguth, Ph.D., the world's foremost psychologist in fetal alcohol disorders.

Ann Streissguth doesn't just speak, she bounces across the stage, imitating a mother rat just slightly brain-damaged by alcohol, doomed to be a careless parent. She dazzles us with her knowledge, compassion and wit. Her blue eyes flash as she teaches the audience the meaning of the word *teratogen*—a substance that causes birth defects.

She explains that what we usually think of as birth defects are such things as missing fingers or toes, or a cleft palate. "But some teratogens, like alcohol, can also cause brain damage, and that's birth defects of the brain. And the brain is what mainly influences behaviour, and that's where we get the behavioural disabilities that are associated with fetal alcohol syndrome and the whole spectrum of disorders that alcohol causes."

> **teratology** . . . 1. A discourse or narrative concerning prodigies; a marvellous tale . . . 2. *Biol.* The study of monstrosities or abnormal formations in animals or plants.
>
> *The Shorter Oxford English Dictionary*

Earlier, the University of Washington's "Teris" website had told me that a teratogen is "an agent that can produce a permanent abnormality of structure or function in an organism exposed during embryonic or fetal life." I'd gone to my heavy, two-volume *Oxford English Dictionary,* and couldn't find *teratogen.* I did find *teratogenesis,* "the production of monsters and misshapen organisms" and a derivation for the term *teratology,* from the Greek word meaning "marvel, prodigy, monster."

The *OED* had it right. Colette could be both a marvel and a monster—sometimes both of these creatures within the same hour. She was not a demon angel, but a cherub whose wings and brain had been damaged before she was born. Colette had all of the cognitive and behavioural characteristics of fetal alcohol effects, and as well, she had been removed from her original nest at eight months of age because of her birth parents' alcoholism. Why had no professional ever seriously looked at fetal alcohol effects as the cause of Colette's problems?

By the time we hit Ann Arbor in November 1997, I had been researching fetal alcohol syndrome (FAS) and fetal alcohol effects (FAE) for eight months—sometimes feeling as if I had been dumped into the icy waters of the Atlantic. The day after the television show, I'd tracked down Dr. Christine Loock, the Vancouver specialist who had diagnosed Jean-François LePage and Mark Steeves, the young men featured on CBC-TV. Agreeing that Colette's learning problems, behaviour and family history were symptomatic of fetal alcohol effects, she gave me a list of people and organizations to call. Following her suggestions, I hit the phone, downloaded material from countless websites and borrowed books from the library.

I also joined the international online support group, FASlink, then sponsored by the Canadian Centre on Substance Abuse (CCSA), and was met by about a hundred messages per day. There were around four hundred correspondents from across North America, and others from Europe, Australia and South Africa—adoptive and foster parents, professionals, and several birth mothers in recovery. Although many were parents of children with full-blown FAS, far more disabled than Colette, others had children who had been diagnosed with FAE and shared similar learning and behaviour problems. Many, like me, had learned about fetal alcohol syndrome through the media (almost never through professionals), and were seeking diagnoses for their children. There were also two adult survivors, both in their forties.

My research indicated that Colette's minor health problems—heart murmur, earaches, slight scoliosis—were consistent with fetal alcohol damage. So were her wide-spaced eyes; cute upturned nose; pronounced overbite (which had been blamed on thumbsucking); downy body hair as a small child; and delays in learning bladder control. Colette's indifference to pain and extremes of temperature, her craving for sweet and fatty foods and early affinity for the "buzz" of alcohol and drugs were possible signals of damaged receptors in the brain. As if to compensate,

41

Mother Nature has given many alcohol-affected people—Colette included—an engaging personality, excellent verbal skills that mask their disabilities and a seemingly spiritual connection with animals.

Historic Warnings

I learned that there have been warnings of the dangers of alcohol to the fetus since Biblical times, when an Old Testament writer urged, "Behold, thou shalt conceive and bear a son: and now drink no wine or strong drinks" (Judges 13:7). Aristotle noted that "foolish, drunken and harebrained women most often bring forth children like unto themselves, morose and languid." The effects of prenatal drinking were also noted in a report by the College of Physicians to the British Parliament in 1726, and in the British House of Commons, in 1834, where a member remarked that infants born to alcoholic mothers sometimes "had a starved, shrivelled and imperfect look."[1]

At the end of the nineteenth century, Dr. William Sullivan, a physician in the Liverpool prison, published a study of 120 incarcerated female "drunkards," noting that their pregnancies often ended in still-births or infant deaths. Several other studies in the first half of the twentieth century indicated a link between maternal alcoholism and damaged children, but this research was not widely known, even in the medical community. As I write, in the twenty-first century, despite numerous medical studies that demonstrate the contrary, there are still doctors advising pregnant women that a drink of alcohol per day can't possibly hurt their babies.

Ground-Breaking Research

In 1968 in Nantes, France, Dr. Paul Lemoine and associates described 127 children born to alcoholic mothers, all exhibiting similar behaviour problems, growth deficiencies and physical anomalies, and published these findings in the French medical journal, *Ouest Medical*. Independently, researchers in Seattle, Washington, were making similar discoveries. While studying infants with "failure to thrive," Dr. Christy Ulleland, a pediatric resident at King County Hospital, noted that all of the children in her study had been born to alcoholic mothers. Dr. David W. Smith, a dysmorphologist (a medical specialist in the study of birth defects) who followed up on Dr. Ulleland's research, examined a little boy from the study, and was struck by the child's short "palpebral fissures" (eye slits). Dr. Smith asked to see the other children of alcoholic mothers, and brought in another dysmorphologist, Dr. Kenneth Lyons Jones. Identifying four more mentally disabled children who shared growth deficiencies and numerous odd facial features, they knew they had made an important medical discovery.

In 1972 the clinical psychologist Ann Streissguth was invited to participate in further research by Jones and Smith. By now, the dysmorphologists had identified eleven unrelated children from three racial backgrounds whose facial features, growth deficiency and central nervous system dysfunction were similar. All eleven had severe learning and behaviour problems, and all had been born to alcoholic mothers. Jones and Smith named this condition "fetal alcohol syndrome." Fascinated, Streissguth did the performance testing for the groundbreaking article in the British medical journal *The Lancet* in June 1973, titled "Pattern of malformation in offspring of chronic alcoholic mothers," which first defined fetal alcohol syndrome. Ulleland, Smith, Jones and Streissguth studied five girls and three boys, aged from three months to four years—eight of the original eleven children—and their mothers. The women ranged in age from twenty-two to forty; two were suffering from delirium tremens and cirrhosis; another was drunk while giving birth.

The children shared many of the same facial features: short eye slits, epicanthal folds (the flap of skin at the inner corner of the eye seen in people of Asian heritage), odd-looking ears, a flat midface (flat cheekbones), a short upturned nose, a low bridge of nose, a smooth or long philtrum (the groove running between the nose and upper lip), a thin upper lip and a small, underdeveloped chin.

Their physical disabilities included heart defects as severe as congestive heart failure, deformed elbows and fingers, hip dislocations, visual problems, incomplete digestive systems and deformed genitals. Seven of the eight had small head circumferences; all had growth deficiencies and were intellectually delayed. Six had been hospitalized for "failure to thrive." The children lagged far behind in social skills and motor performance. Five of the eight children engaged in "repetitive self-stimulating behaviour such as head rolling, head banging, or rocking."

The *Lancet* study received wide media coverage, and also changed Streissguth's life. Since 1973 she has been involved with countless studies dealing with the effects of alcohol on the fetus; developed prevention programs; and worked at building worldwide awareness. Her studies indicate that "moderate" drinking can do considerable invisible damage to the fetal brain. For example, one ounce of pure alcohol per day in pregnancy (two drinks or ten ounces of wine) can lower the baby's IQ by seven points—possibly the difference between passing and failing high school math.[2] Recent studies indicate that just one occasion of social drinking (four to five drinks) in pregnancy can cause permanent brain damage to the fetus.[3]

Invisible Disabilities

The small, wispy, intellectually impaired children of the original *Lancet* study had little in common with sturdy, quick-witted, athletic Colette. But by the late 1970s researchers at the University of Washington had recognized a large invisible group of alcohol-damaged people—seemingly healthy children and adults with relatively normal intelligence, who nevertheless struggled with neurological injuries caused by prenatal alcohol. The facial characteristics of FAS were minimal, and had often vanished by the mid-teens. These children and adults had normal or slightly below normal scores on the usual IQ tests, but exhibited learning and behaviour problems that indicated dysfunctional central nervous systems, and their mothers had abused alcohol in pregnancy. In 1978 Dr. Sterling Clarren, a diagnostician with the University of Washington, coined the term "fetal alcohol effects" (FAE) now known as alcohol-related neurodevelopmental disorder (ARND).

The Institute of Medicine's 1996 diagnostic criteria for ARND include a history of maternal drinking in pregnancy and ". . . a complex pattern of behaviour or cognitive abnormalities that are inconsistent with developmental level and cannot be explained by familial background or environment alone." The description fit Colette perfectly: learning difficulties, school problems, poor impulse control, poor social perception, deficits in expressive language, poor capacity for abstraction and/or deficits in mathematical skills, memory, attention and judgment.[4]

By the end of the twentieth century, fetal alcohol spectrum disorder (FASD) began to be used as an umbrella term denoting several kinds of diagnosis, just as the word *cancer* can refer to a number of debilitating conditions. Streissguth and others estimate that about 2 in 1,000 individuals in industrialized countries have full-blown FAS, and three to four times this number will have ARND. In other words, about 10 in 1,000—1 in 100—North Americans are likely to have some degree of fetal alcohol damage.[5]

CONFUSING FAS LINGO

Over the years, as research became more sophisticated, the terminology used for fetal alcohol disorders frequently shifted. Here are some of the acronyms and terms on my learning curve:

FAS

Full-blown fetal alcohol syndrome, characterized by small head circumference, various facial features, severely impaired intelligence, possible physical defects and/or behaviour problems and an alcoholic mother who drank very heavily in pregnancy.

ARND

Alcohol-related neurodevelopmental disorder. Individuals may appear normal, and have normal or even above-average intelligence, but may have some of the facial or physical features of FAS, along with learning and behaviour problems, and a history of maternal drinking in pregnancy. Formerly known as FAE (fetal alcohol effects).

pFAS

Partial fetal alcohol syndrome is similar to ARND. Other terms include prenatal exposure to alcohol (PEA) and static encephalopathy—alcohol exposed.

FASD

The new umbrella term that refers to the entire spectrum of fetal alcohol disorders, formerly known as FAS/FAE or FAS/E.

ADHD

Attention deficit hyperactivity disorder. A frequent but rarely helpful diagnosis for people affected by prenatal alcohol. The usual medication for ADHD is Ritalin, which is often not effective in children with FASD.

Teratogen

A substance that causes permanent birth defects. Alcohol is a teratogen. Other well-known teratogens are thalidomide, codeine, toluene and dilantin. Coffee, tobacco, marijuana, heroin and cocaine may temporarily affect infants but are not considered to be teratogens.

Primary disabilities

The learning and behaviour problems resulting from fetal alcohol damage.

Secondary disabilities

The behaviour problems in individuals with FASD, resulting when family, schools and community fail to understand or support their primary, organic, disabilities.

Frightening Statistics

Studying the long-term effects of FAS along with those of the seemingly milder ARND (then known as FAE), Streissguth learned that prenatal alcohol damage that was previously thought to be slight can actually be a pernicious neurological impairment that lasts a lifetime. She found that those apparently normal individuals at the high-functioning end of the spectrum—people like Colette—fare *worse* in life than people with the obvious mental disabilities of full-blown FAS, because they are brighter, *invisibly* disabled, seldom diagnosed or given adequate support and more difficult to control.

I was stunned by her 1996 longitudinal study with the unwieldy title *Understanding the Occurrence of Secondary Disabilities in Clients with Fetal Alcohol Syndrome (FAS) and Fetal Alcohol Effects (FAE)*. Mainly consisting of simple but dramatic bar graphs, the seventy-one-page study looks at 473 clients ranging in age from three to fifty-one—178 with FAS and an average IQ of 79; 295 with FAE and an average IQ of 90.

Streissguth's study clearly links FASD with "secondary disabilities": dropping out of school early, addiction and alcoholism, trouble with the law, unemployment, sexual offences, difficulties in living independently, lack of parenting skills and mental illness. Sixty percent of the children studied had been diagnosed with attention deficit hyperactivity disorder (ADHD). And between the ages of twelve and fifty-one,

- 94 percent of the interviewees had been diagnosed with a mental health disorder;
- 60 percent had experienced confinement in a mental institution, drug or alcohol rehabilitation facility or prison;
- 60 percent had disrupted school experience (dropping out, expulsion or suspension);
- 60 percent had experienced trouble with the law;
- 50 percent had demonstrated inappropriate sexual behaviour;

- 50 percent had alcohol and drug problems;
- 80 percent had problems with both employment and independent living.

Of the clients over the age of twenty-one,

- 50 percent had been diagnosed with depression;
- 30 percent reported hearing voices or seeing visions;
- 23 percent had attempted suicide.

The study also indicates that alcohol-affected individuals have great difficulty parenting. Twenty-eight percent of females over age twelve and 10 percent of the males had become parents—one becoming a parent at only thirteen. Forty percent of the women had drunk alcohol during pregnancy: the majority of these babies had suffered prenatal alcohol damage and were not being raised by their parents.

The Aboriginal Tragedy

I learned that in North America the incidence of FASD is highest in aboriginal communities, both rural and urban; among African-Americans; and among people of low socio-economic status. Full-blown FAS, complete with small head size, severe developmental delays and often physical defects, is not unusual among Canada's aboriginal people, and is also common among Native Americans and "Aleuts" in the United States. A large-scale birth defects monitoring program at the Center for Disease Control in the United States found that Native Americans have a rate of FAS more than thirty-two times that of whites, while African-Americans are more than six times as likely to have FAS as white Americans.

The tragic results of maternal alcoholism among Native Americans were documented in the late Michael Dorris's ground-breaking 1989 book, *The Broken Cord*. The book tells the story of his adopted son Abel (called Adam in the book), who struggled with FAS throughout his short and painful life. In 1991, shortly before the book was produced as a film, Abel, then twenty-three, died after being hit by a car. When interviewed by Dorris for his book, the Lakota activist Elaine Boudreau told him that at least a third of the population of any school system on her Minnesota reserve had emotional and learning problems and histories of family alcohol use that were consistent with a diagnosis of fetal alcohol damage.

In 1997 three University of Manitoba researchers—Dr. Ab Chudley, a geneticist; Dr. Michael Moffatt, a pediatrician; and a graduate student, Debra Kowlessar—were invited to study the children in an aboriginal community in rural Manitoba after teachers complained that half of the reserve's children were incapable of learning. The study indicated alcohol exposure in 46 percent of the mothers of the 179 children assessed. Eighteen of those children—10 percent of those studied—were found to have some physical signs of FAS or partial FAS (pFAS) and were diagnosed accordingly. Dr. Chudley told me that although the alcohol-exposed children without any physical features were not formally identified, he believes that another 20 to 30 percent probably show some learning and behaviour impairment as well.

The massive Canadian Royal Commission Report on Aboriginal Peoples, published in 1995, heard testimony from social workers and others working with FAS in aboriginal communities:

> FAS causes particularly acute pain among Aboriginal people—the pain of accepting responsibility for having caused harm. This is the dilemma facing a woman whose drinking has damaged her children and the community that allowed it to happen. . . .

Kim Meawasige, a socal worker who has worked with numerous aboriginal street youth in Toronto, gave me an even more tragic testimony. She told me of a photo from a teen camp she had organized around 1995, which showed four beaming native fifteen-year-olds—two male, two female—just enjoying the beach. Six years later, all were dead.

One was thrown off a balcony, one was beaten to death, one was burned to death, one was murdered horribly. All of them had been adopted but had wound up in numerous foster and group homes. All had trouble with the law, trouble on the street, and some of them "worked on the street." And I'm convinced all of them had undiagnosed FAS.

"Stack Attack Victims"

Donna Debolt, a former FAS specialist with the government of Alberta, confirms the high numbers of children with FASD in foster care. She participated in a government investigation in southern Alberta, a region with a total population of 146,000. All children in care of child protection services were assessed for fetal alcohol damage, and 50 percent were found to have FASD. Among children in permanent care and thus available for adoption, 70 percent had FASD.

For more than twenty years Debolt has fought hard for children in care, and has coined a phrase describing the most damaged ones: *stack attack victims.* "This means that if anything could go wrong for a child it did—prenatal alcohol exposure, abuse, neglect, multiple foster homes, adoption breakdowns, school disruption (following inappropriate school 'plans'), trouble with the law and basically nobody who cares! That last point is frequently seen with children of the 'system.' *Can you believe there are children in this world who have nobody who lights up when they come into the room?*" She adds that the phenomenon of stack attack creates unending dilemmas for diagnosticians, who often fail to recognize the first assault on the child—that of prenatal alcohol before he was born.

Trouble with the Law

Given the learning problems, poor judgment, impulsiveness and addictiveness of most people with FASD, we shouldn't be surprised that many wind up in the criminal justice system. Streissguth's secondary disabilities study indicates that two-thirds of males with FASD over the age of twelve will have trouble with the law, and more than half of those involved with the law will be convicted.

Donna Debolt has developed programs for young offenders in Alberta and told me that at least 25 percent of young repeat offenders probably have FASD. "Those numbers could go as high as 50 percent or more for 'stack attack' inmates, that core of repeat offenders who got in trouble young, stayed in trouble and have experienced school disruption, mental health issues, homelessness and joblessness."

After the Aha! Moment

Donna Debolt describes what she calls the Aha! moment, when parents suddenly see that FASD could be the explanation that has eluded them. They generally re-examine their child's past and, for the first time, everything fits.

In 1983, when we adopted cute, bouncy, bright, three-year-old Colette, we knew nothing about fetal alcohol damage. In the care of a loving foster family since the age of eight months, she had seemed physically and mentally healthy, despite that "ventricular septal defect" (heart murmur), which I now know is common among children with FASD. Children's Aid Society never hinted that her birth mother's drinking in pregnancy might result in learning difficulties and behaviour problems at a later age.

The "non-identifying information" we had received about Colette's biological mother, indicated that at the age of twelve, "Harriet" had been abandoned by her own mother, who died a few years later. Remaining with her alcoholic father, Harriet quickly became addicted to alcohol. She went on to bear three children by two fathers, and all were removed from her care. This history indicates that Harriet, too, may have been affected by prenatal alcohol. As the Institute of Medicine textbook notes:

Alcohol is usual in the family of birth of women who drink during pregnancy; early experimentation with alcohol is common; first pregnancy often occurs at a very young age; FAS and other levels of alcohol-related damage usually occur in later pregnancies and in the later years of childbearing; child neglect is frequent; unstable domestic relations are common . . . there is a general lack of stable employment . . . and low education and unstable living conditions are frequent. Commonly, there is intervention by others with the children after birth to protect them from chaotic home environments.[6]

Streissguth's study indicates that unlike the primary damage of prenatal alcohol, secondary disabilities result because families and communities generally fail to provide the support and structure required by a person with FASD. For example, with the structure provided by the Hincks Treatment Centre, which we were unable to duplicate, Colette could do very well. Without this support, her poor judgment, impulsiveness and other learning problems resulted in a downward spiral from one disaster to another.

As I looked over Streissguth's suggestions for prevention of secondary disabilities, I remembered the summer day when I looked out on the front veranda and saw four-year-old Colette perched at the top of a flower box, four feet up, holding giant fern fronds and furiously flapping her arms. When Cleo, who was six, and her eight-year-old buddy Melissa felt she was flapping fast enough, they yelled, "Jump!" and she leapt off, expecting to fly, but instead landing on the ground with a thud. Dismayed, she got to her feet and brushed off the dirt. "You nearly did it," they urged. "This time, flap harder!" So she picked up the fern fronds, climbed back onto the flower box, and flapped and jumped and thudded again—until I interrupted their little game and took her inside for cookies and ice cream. Was Cleo being malicious, or did she honestly believe her sister could fly?

I realized that since first grade, Colette's family, schools and community had expected her to fly. Professional after professional said that she should flap harder, or that if Brian and I improved our parenting skills, she wouldn't hit the ground with a thud. With tears of rage and frustration, Colette tried to explain that she *couldn't* fly, but nobody understood. Eventually she stopped flapping her wings altogether, and sought comfort in sex, drugs and heavy metal music.

Colette, by the age of seventeen, had struggled with *every one* of those secondary disabilities, except parenting problems. Her many fine qualities—physical beauty and strength, intelligence, sense of humour, charm, fun-loving personality, talent for working with animals—seemed to have gone to waste. Despite our best efforts, she was a school dropout, sexually promiscuous, addictive, seemingly unemployable and homeless. She had been involved with the law, incarcerated for two years in a psychiatric treatment centre, and diagnosed with conduct disorder and oppositional defiant disorder. She had never become pregnant because of my diligence in taking her for quarterly shots of Depo Provera (a highly effective progesterone-based contraceptive that is injected every three months).

Brian and I thought of ourselves as well informed: we subscribed to two daily newspapers, read numerous magazines and watched public affairs television. But until that TV show, despite all our trips to doctors and therapists, only my friend Keitha, recovering from alcoholism, had suggested that Colette might be struggling with fetal alcohol damage.

I now sense that both professionals and the general public mistakenly believe that only children of aboriginal ancestry are affected by pre-natal alcohol. If Colette had been a little girl of Mohawk or Inuit heritage, instead of a tall blond child of Anglo-Saxon background, with a vocabulary and grammar developed in a well-educated family of non-stop talkers, her condition might have been more obvious.

It's probable that when we adopted Colette in 1983, five years after the University of Washington researchers recognized those nearly invisible fetal alcohol effects, this information had not spread to Toronto. Still, Streissguth's statistics indicate that if we had known of the possibility of fetal alcohol damage when we adopted her at age three, we might have prevented many of those secondary disabilities and changed the course of her life.

FAS-Coloured Glasses

Put on your fetal alcohol glasses. You'll see that every time you read the newspaper, cases will jump out that are pure fetal alcohol. The welfare mother who starves her baby to death, the kid who shoots his brother, the sex offender, the repeat offender who hangs herself in prison—most of them are suffering brain damage caused by a mother who drank.

—MARGARET SPRENGER, FASD ADVOCATE

If one out of every one hundred North Americans is living with FASD, I realized, I must know some. I began thinking about people I knew whose odd behaviour could have been caused by prenatal alcohol damage. In my own large extended family, there were several distant relations whose behaviour had been bizarre since birth. They had problems in school, lied, stole, dropped out of school at an early age, became addicted to alcohol or drugs, lived on the fringes of society.

One is the son of a delightful, extroverted couple who loved parties—born about seven months after his father set off to World War II. It's not hard to imagine: a loving couple about to be separated by a cataclysmic war, wondering if they would see each other again, nights of farewell parties, other, later nights, when a lonely pregnant woman struggled with fear, loss and pain. Who could link those evenings of rye whiskey and ginger ale with a son who had problems in school, could never be trusted, had frequent encounters with the law and was eventually disowned by his sorrowing parents?

In the middle-class academic community where I grew up, some families had children whose behaviour was the target of much gossip. Could those frequent Saturday night parties, at which alcohol flowed, though nobody got drunk, have been connected with the dropout teenage daughter whose delinquency and promiscuity shocked the neighbourhood? Or those three brats whose learning and behaviour problems puzzled their loving parents, both of whom had Ph.D.s? FAS had not yet been discovered. Could a few social drinks each Saturday night have caused some of these problems?

In our daughters' upscale elementary school of four hundred pupils, the numerical estimate arrived at by Streissguth and other researchers—one in one hundred—might indicate there were four children with fetal alcohol damage, three in addition to Colette. But I could recall at least eight possibilities in our daughters' special education classes. Among them was the handsome son of a single mother on welfare, an Artful Dodger with no conscience, who lived by his wits and dropped out of school in sixth grade. There was a large, heavy boy who terrified Cleo with his bullying. Then there was the tiny, waifish girl with both visual and hearing difficulties (often symptomatic of FASD): she was daughter of professionals who had divorced while the mother was pregnant, quite possibly drowning her sorrows, along with her baby, in alcohol. Of the two dozen "emotionally disturbed" teenagers who had been at the Hincks farm with Colette, at least half shared her constellation of learning and behaviour problems, along with family backgrounds that indicated possible maternal drinking.

Monitoring the newspapers, I spotted the possible FAS stories. Throughout April 1997, the local media covered the inquest into the tragic homicide of a twenty-three-month-old toddler, whose crack addict mother had starved and beaten her to death in 1993, despite warnings to the Children's Aid Society from the child's former foster mother. Christie Blatchford of the *Toronto Sun* wrote of the autopsy photographs, which showed a baby who was "utterly emaciated, visibly bruised and battered on every inch of her wasted frame." Blatchford described the mother as "oafish," with a "cat smile"; a "belligerent lump" who "clearly . . . does not feel guilty."

After the mother's trial in 1994, she was sentenced to a four-year term for manslaughter. The presiding judge told her, "I am not at all persuaded that you have come to accept the gravity and seriousness of your crime."[7] Her lack of remorse, addictiveness, string of criminal offences, inability to parent and family history of alcoholism and drug addiction strongly pointed to a mother who had been damaged before birth, and who exhibited every single one of Ann Streissguth's secondary disabilities.

Observing the newspaper photos of possible "invisible FASD" stories, I noticed that numerous male offenders had similar faces—slightly triangular or long in shape, with many of the following features: prominent forehead and receding hairline; wide-spaced eyes; low bridge of nose; low-set or odd-shaped ears; underdeveloped chin. Nearly all wore moustaches, possibly to cover the lack of philtrum, the notch that most of us have on our upper lip. (A flat upper lip is almost always a sign of fetal alcohol damage.) Key words that indicated a strong possibility of prenatal alcohol damage began to jump out at me, often describing defendants in criminal trials:

- slight build
- receding jaw
- quiet
- unresponsive
- seeming lack of remorse
- model prisoner
- learning disabled
- ADHD
- unemployed
- welfare recipient
- violent rages
- alcoholic
- addict
- school dropout
- repeat offender
- alcoholic parents or broken home
- native background
- foster child
- adopted

The Invisible Tragedy

*Nobody really knows the full cost of caring for the FASD
population, and there must be a wide range depending on
adaptive abilities. That is, the range would be very expensive
to unbelievably expensive! Once you get to numbers in the
millions, I don't think anybody really believes them even
though they are true.*

—DR. STERLING CLARREN (CORRESPONDENCE
WITH AUTHOR)

If the estimates are correct, about 3 million Americans and 300,000
Canadians can never live up to their genetic potential, because of prenatal alcohol. Yet no large-scale economic study in recent years has
investigated the financial price of FASD to society, partly because
most alcohol-affected individuals are never identified. The amount
spent to support them is buried in government accounts: extra
medicare for various birth defects; special education; mental health;
addictions; criminal justice; and social services such as subsidized
housing, welfare and disability support. A 1985 study by Henrick
Harwood and Diane Napolitano, American economic analysts, estimated the lifetime direct and indirect costs of medical and social
services for an individual with FAS as $596,000.[8] A 1989 report by
Johne [sic] Binkley of the Alaska State Senate indicated that the lifetime cost of each individual with FASD is about $1.4 million (around
$2 million in current dollars). This report looked only at medical and
social costs: these numbers do not include the costs of welfare, the
justice system, mild physical problems, mild learning disabilities or
loss of a useful member of society.[9]

Closer to home, H. Philip Hepworth, an advisor for Canada's
National Crime Prevention Strategy, outlined the cost of a typical
young offender from birth to age 17. The child of dysfunctional alcoholic parents, "Jack" first comes into contact with social services before

his first birthday, and displays developmental problems before age three. Taken into protective custody at six, he spends five years in a series of foster homes; is placed in a group home at eleven because of his "acting-out" behaviour; and has "trouble with the law" before his twelfth birthday. Although Jack is not described as having FASD, his alcoholic parents and developmental delays make his situation classic. Before his eighteenth birthday, he costs the taxpayers $511,000 for psychological and psychiatric care, "special needs" child care, special education, foster and group home care, social workers, various court cases and one year of closed custody.[10]

In her 2003 doctoral thesis, Toronto researcher Brenda Stade, assisted by economist Wendy Ungar, estimated that children and youth with FASD under the age of 21 cost our nation around $344 million annually. The researchers looked only at the extra costs of health care, education, social services and loss of productivity. They did not include costs of criminal justice in this age group.[11]

Given Colette's own costs to the Canadian taxpayer for the first 24 years of her life, I believe that the $2 million lifetime estimate for an alcohol-affected person might be conservative. But we cannot put a price on the tragic waste of worldwide human potential: how many great artists, athletes, musicians, entertainers, thinkers has our world lost to prenatal alcohol?

The incidence in Eastern Europe and Russia seems to be even higher. FASlink correspondents in South Africa, Australia, Germany and New Zealand indicate similar problems, and equal ignorance on the part of the medical profession and governments. Apart from a handful of activists and medical researchers, few have taken the trouble to make the link between maternal drinking and the profound, preventable, permanent disability suffered by millions of people worldwide. The majority of North American professionals—teachers, school administrators, doctors, psychiatrists, psychologists, lawyers, judges, social workers—have never bothered to read any of the thousands of academic studies about prenatal alcohol, or to attend the conferences on FASD that are held frequently on both sides of the U.S.–Canada border.

Listening to Ann Streissguth in that first conference in Ann Arbor, I had no idea of the journey I was beginning, or that I would have the privilege of interviewing her twice. A battle-scarred advocate for people with FASD, she created the international newsletter *Iceberg* in 1991, forging a coalition of the University of Washington's Fetal Alcohol and Drug Unit, the university's diagnostic clinic, parents and other concerned professionals:

> To me, the metaphor 'Iceberg' has two meanings. One is, we see those people that have the clear physical features but we don't identify those others who have primarily the Central Nervous System abnormality. But even one [alcohol-affected] person is an iceberg. The part you see doesn't really identify the part that's going to have the problem. Very few of the children need oral surgery for example, but they all need some kind of help with their central nervous system problems. (Telephone interview with author, 2001.)

What I learned on that 1997 learning curve turned my world upside down. I realized that in the industrialized world, a large proportion of those countless people living on the fringes of society are not there because they have inferior genes. They are not inherently lazy, stupid or evil—although their learning and behaviour problems make them appear that way. The root of the problem is not childhood neglect or abuse although for many, disruptive families have compounded their problems. They live in self-perpetuating ignorance, poverty and crime because they came into the world with permanent neurological damage that could have been prevented. Most are never diagnosed, and when their specific problems and needs are not addressed,

- adoption into loving homes often cannot help them;
- Head Start programs are often ineffective in helping learning and behaviour problems;

- special education and behaviour programs in school frequently cannot help them;
- traditional psychotherapy approaches rarely work;
- the usual twelve-step approach to addiction and alcoholism is unlikely to be effective; and
- existing prisons and penitentiaries can do little more than warehouse criminal offenders with FASD keeping them from committing crimes until they are released.

Every piece of information I received led me to two inescapable conclusions. First, very little of what we had tried in the fourteen years since we had adopted Colette could possibly have worked. Our attempts were doomed because none of the dozens of professionals we had consulted—doctors, teachers, psychologists, social workers, psychiatrists—had the foggiest idea that we were dealing with *permanent brain damage caused by prenatal alcohol.* Instead of helping us find strategies appropriate to her neurological problems, they either blamed her for her bad behaviour, or blamed us for our bad parenting.

My second conclusion: our story is not an isolated case, and our daughter is not alone in her complex, misunderstood disability. On the contrary, she is just one small person among the damaged millions worldwide, all stranded on the colossal iceberg that costs the taxpayers billions and leaves generations of tragic individuals struggling in its wake.

The "iceberg" is fetal alcohol spectrum disorder.

CHAPTER FOUR

Diagnosis: An Excuse for Bad Behaviour?

There is a myth that if a child is not accurately diagnosed, he or she will not be labelled. But family after family comes into my office and shows me report cards, pre-sentence reports, and court judgments that label. The labels used are hurtful. They include "Lazy, stupid, does not try, poorly motivated, psychopath."

A diagnosis of FAS or FAE usually ends the moral labels so loved by schools and courts. A diagnosis . . . should not be used to close doors, but rather to open them wider, by making modifications in programs to accommodate special needs, by adding to the understanding that teachers, social workers, lawyers and judges have for affected individuals.

Affected adolescents tell me over and over again that a diagnosis helped them because teachers, parents and others saw them in a different way. "Now they say my brain is different, they don't call me stupid any more," is a common remark that I hear.

—Dr. Jo Nanson, neuropsychologist, Saskatoon

The trip to Ann Arbor in November 1997 convinced Brian and me that we were on the right track. It had been a rough year. Since February, despite Colette's special supported classroom, she had once again fallen into stealing, truancy and addiction, and only another Hincks Farm could have prevented the crash that followed.

Cleo, too, was having problems. Her learning difficulties, seasonal affective disorder and distractable nature (later diagnosed as ADHD) made it almost impossible for her to concentrate. She'd dropped out of high school and had gone through a series of dead-end jobs. She had a new boyfriend who was unemployed and frequently abusive—and she seemed powerless to break up with him.

Having accepted an early retirement package, Brian started a second career as a personal coach, and our financial situation remained precarious as he tried to get established. I was working on a screenplay with a partner, and in the evenings hit the Internet to continue my FAS research. We worked hard at supporting each other—lots of hugs, jokes, little treats—but sometimes we seemed to be slogging through sticky porridge.

In May 1997, on the recommendation of Vancouver's Dr. Christine Loock (who had diagnosed the two young men I'd seen on TV), I called the Toronto Hospital for Sick Children's Motherisk Clinic, asking them to assess Colette for FAE. The intake worker told me that the clinic did not diagnose adolescents over the age of sixteen, that I should have had this done many years earlier. I recalled, but didn't mention, taking Colette to this hospital at age ten, begging for help, and having been told she was "normal." The worker didn't know anyone else in Ontario who could do a diagnosis. On Dr. Loock's suggestion, I called one of the clinic's doctors. "Why is a diagnosis so important to you?" she asked, bewildered. "There's nothing that can be done anyway."

I wondered if the doctors in the hospital's cancer ward would hesitate to diagnose a child's leukemia or brain tumour, because "nothing can be done." The Streissguth study talked of "protective factors" that would prevent or reduce the secondary disabilities caused by fetal alcohol. The second most important protective factor is diagnosis before the age of six. But in 1983 one of my FASlink friends, Stephen Neafcy, had been diagnosed with FAE at forty-three. He wrote of the great relief he felt at learning that his school problems, impulsiveness, inappropriate sexual behaviours and gambling addiction were the result of prenatal neurological damage:

> My problem was not knowing I was FAE until age 43. I was expected to fly with the flock when I had a broken wing! Using this broken wing to try to glide with all my peers was a living hell but the worst was failing and seeing the disappointment in Mom and Dad's eyes . . . (Stephen Neafcy, living with FAE, from a post to FASlink, 1999)

By May 1997 Colette was back to her old habits: vanishing on weekends, skipping a great deal of school and, despite family efforts at security, stealing money for drugs at every opportunity. Knowing there was nothing more Brian and I could do to protect her, I felt burned out and afraid for her safety, obsessed by those dozens of e-mails I read every morning and evening.

A friend who had been widowed two years previously suggested a grief therapist who lived in the next block. Slim, blond, luminous Dr. Lynne Thurling had raised four children as a single mother, and is a psychiatrist experienced in both addiction and neurological trauma. For the better part of a year, I sat in her cheerful study late each Wednesday afternoon, leaving after an hour feeling that I could survive yet another week.

Summer 1997. The downward spiral continued. Colette moved into an apartment over a pool hall with her thirty-seven-year-old boyfriend, "Dennis," and an older couple, all alcoholics and drug users. The building was a notorious hot-bed of prostitution and crack dealers. Colette told me that Dennis was of native background, adopted into a wealthy family: I wondered if his adoptive parents were feeling as exhausted and desperate as Brian and I. Many of our friends advised us to sever our relationship with her, but instead we tried to stay in contact with her, encouraging her to phone us, trying to meet her for lunch once a week. Knowing that any money we gave her would be spent on drugs, we gave her only bus tokens.

Colette had always been a little on the heavy side, but now had lost about thirty pounds and looked gaunt and ravaged. On one of our occasional trips to her favourite burger joint, I told her a little about the research I was doing. "I feel really bad," I said. "I think that all of the problems you've had all your life are not really your fault." She was intrigued.

I talked to her about all the times we had listened to teachers say she could do better, and she had sat there crying because she was doing the best she could. She'd been diagnosed with learning disabilities, but nobody had realized how hard it was for her to pay attention for long periods of time, or to finish her work. "You're not bad or stupid. Dad and I think that the real problem could be, you have a tiny bit of brain damage because your birth mom drank when she was pregnant with you."

"You mean I'm crazy?"

"No, you're not crazy. I've got head problems too—those awful migraines. And what about Cleo—something's wrong with her brain chemistry so that she gets depressed in winter. In fact, you're so smart that nobody ever figured out that you could have these problems." Glugging the end of her milkshake, she told me the people at her apartment were out of milk and asked to "borrow" four dollars. I knew it was for cigarettes but gave it to her anyway.

In early August, overwhelmed and exhausted, we spent a few days at our cabin, having ordered Cleo not to tell Colette we were away, and not to let her into our house. But Colette persuaded her sister to allow her to print some resumés in my office, then rummaged through the desk drawers and stole a chequebook. She then wrote six cheques to herself for a total of $2,000, forged my signature and managed to cash them at her own bank. Several days later, I tried to get cash from a bank machine and found that my checking account had been drained.

This was the third time she had committed bank fraud. At thirteen, she had forged withdrawal slips on Cleo's bank account, emptying it of the entire $100. And the previous October, she had slipped my Interac card from my wallet and withdrawn $50 from my account, guessing that I had stupidly used my telephone pass code as my PIN number.

My bank tracked down the cheques, all badly forged. I was furious with her, and terrified to the point that I thought she'd be *safer* in a detention centre. The bank refunded my money and wouldn't press charges. The fraud squad weren't interested, even though she had confessed to committing the forgery. The drug squad didn't care that a thirty-five-year-old man was supplying a seventeen-year-old with alcohol, marijuana and probably crack. The vice squad knew that the apartments over the pool hall housed numerous prostitutes, but did not care what an addicted teenager might be doing with her body in return for the drugs which kept her wired and weird. Desperate, I lied to Colette, telling her that she risked going to jail if she didn't get rehab, because I was going to press charges. Admitting she was addicted to crack, she spent ten days in a detox centre for women, while I tried to find a rehab program that would take her.

She needed far more than the three-week program offered by government-supported agencies, and most would not accept females under the age of eighteen. I found two private rehab centres offering three-month programs for $30,000, which we couldn't afford. Finally, I tracked down a government-supported six-month residential coeducational program for young adults aged sixteen to twenty, two hundred miles away. This facility agreed to admit her, but couldn't give me a date. So Colette came home from detox to wait for admission, spending her time sleeping and watching TV.

The Sealed File Barrier

A FASlink friend suggested I try getting a diagnosis from "Dr. Brown," a geneticist outside Toronto who occasionally diagnosed FAS. I booked an appointment for October 6, several months away. Now I had to get Colette to come with me. And knowing that her birth parents were alcoholics wasn't enough: to get the diagnosis we needed to know how much her birth mother had drunk in pregnancy. This meant opening a lot of sealed files.

The non-identifying information provided to Colette by CAS back in 1994 said only that in August 1980, "You came into care . . . following concerns by neighbours that you were not being properly cared for or supervised." The information also indicated that by 1982, "the agency was concerned that your birth family was not able to change their lifestyle and provide a home for you and were considering asking that you be made a Crown Ward allowing you to be placed for adoption." I told Colette that a diagnosis could mean some government financial support down the way, and she agreed to cooperate in whatever way she could.

I phoned my next-door neighbour, Terry. An adoptive mother herself, she worked in the non-identifying disclosure department for the Children's Aid Society. I asked her how I could learn about Colette's birth mother's drinking habits in pregnancy. She told me that if I wrote her a letter she could search the CAS files. She also explained that the Adoption Disclosure Register of Ontario, another provincial government office, holds the files of every adoption in the province and will unite birth parents and adoptees over the age of eighteen, provided both have registered. The register will also do searches for adult adoptees who want to track down a member of their birth family—but the backlog is now about seven years. However, she said, if we could request an emergency search for medical reasons, we could speed things up.

Dear Ms Kent,
I support the request of my Mom, Bonnie Buxton, to have a search for my birth father's parents and my brother. I really need to know if my birth mother drank while she was pregnant with me. (Letter from Colette to Ontario Adoption Disclosure Registry, August 20, 1997)

Enclosing Colette's letter, I wrote to the Ontario Adoption Disclosure Registry, requesting an emergency search for her paternal grandmother, on medical grounds. CAS's non-identifying information indicated that this hard-working woman had raised Colette's full brother, two years older, when the family broke down. I hoped she could tell me about her daughter-in-law's drinking habits in pregnancy. Our family doctor wrote a letter backing up the medical need for this search. We also wrote letters to Terry at CAS requesting a search of Colette's files. Terry quickly followed up, but could not find any additional information.

By early September Colette was again ignoring curfew. Even worse, she had found the hidden strongbox for my parent support group and had taken about three hundred dollars—leaving only a five-dollar bill. I told her to pack her bag, and drove her to the police station, where she admitted to ripping me off. When I told the officer at the desk that I wanted to press charges, he told us to sit in a corner and wait until the appropriate officer came back from dinner.

I looked at her, hunched over, tears in her eyes, bleak and desperate. I didn't have the energy to go through the lengthy court battle we'd gone through three years earlier. I couldn't afford it, either. Back in 1994, the lawyer's bill of about $1,000 had been paid by legal aid. Now the provincial government had eliminated legal aid for young offenders, so Brian and I would have to pay. Even more important, I was now certain that her actions were the result of prenatal brain damage, made worse by a society that was ignorant of a disorder that was filling our special education classrooms and our jails. Moreover, I'd disobeyed one of the key rules of my support group: if your child steals from you, lock up your valuables securely. But I couldn't live with this turmoil one more day, and neither could Brian or Cleo. "Come on, Colette," I said. "I'll drive you to a shelter."

On Monday, September 8, 1997, I received a lengthy form from the Adoption Disclosure Register, regarding our request for an emergency medical search, which needed to be filled out by the diagnosing physician. The letter written by our family doctor, outlining our family's struggle with Colette, and the probability of undiagnosed fetal alcohol damage, was not enough. The diagnosing physician was asked to indicate whether a diagnosis could result in preventive treatment, and if so, what kind of treatment. But the doctor at Sick Children's Hospital had told me nothing could be done for FAS.

Nevertheless, a diagnosis might give us an answer to the question: *Why have things gone so terribly wrong with Colette?* It might allow us to move forward, build some other kind of relationship with her—what kind of relationship, I didn't know. Dismayed, I threw the form on top of the stack on my in-basket.

Three days later, a worker at the Children's Aid Society answered a phone call from a distraught woman. She needed to find her biological niece, who had been taken into the care of the CAS in infancy and adopted at age three. Several months earlier, the girl's father had written to the CAS, asking them to find her, as her grandmother had terminal cancer. CAS never responded. Now, the dying grandmother was unlikely to last the weekend. Her last wish was to see her missing granddaughter—Colette, who was now seventeen. Could the worker please help?

Ordinarily, a CAS worker would have said that nothing could be done. This was confidential information, she would explain, adding that the child would be free to register with the Adoption Disclosure Register at age eighteen. But amazingly, Colette's aunt had reached the only worker in CAS who knew Colette—had known her since the age of three—my next-door neighbour and fellow adoptive mother who had been attempting to help us find the very grandmother who was now dying. "Yes," said Terry. "I will help you."

That evening, I received an urgent call from a worker at the Adoption Disclosure Register. She told me that Colette's birth family had also requested an emergency search, as Colette's grandmother was dying. Everything came together. Within minutes I was on the phone to Colette's aunt.

Early the following morning, I snapped photos in her grandparents' tiny apartment as Colette met her grandmother—frail and ill, but amazingly alert—along with her grandfather and two aunts. One aunt drove Colette to meet her birth father and full brother "Joey," while her grandfather and remaining aunt gave me tea and cookies, and I gave them photos of Colette growing up. I mentioned some of what we had been going through, and they told me about Colette's birth mother's drinking habits in pregnancy. She had gone on frequent binges of as long as three weeks while she was pregnant with Colette, also chain-smoking and using Valium and marijuana. She'd had odd red spots on her arms, which her doctor had attributed to her alcohol abuse. Later, Colette's birth father confirmed this information.

Lying in a hospital bed in an adjacent alcove in the tiny apartment, Colette's grandmother weakly called out, asking to talk to me. I wish that Colette could have known this wonderful woman when she was well. Photos in the apartment showed a tall, muscular matriarch, evidence of the family height and physical strength that Colette had inherited. Now reduced by cancer to skin and bones, she held my hand and smiled while I told her as many positive or funny stories about Colette as I could muster up. "Thank you for raising her," she said, squeezing my hand. "She's a lovely girl. You've done a wonderful job." I bit my lip and tried not to cry.

Three days later, her grandmother died, and Colette asked for my support at the funeral. Outside the chapel, she introduced me to her biological father and brother, Joey, both over six feet tall. We slid into the back pew and looked around with curiosity at Colette's many aunts, uncles and cousins. The family resemblances were striking. Joey, just two years older than Colette, has identical fair hair, skin and hazel eyes: he and Colette could be twins. Colette remains in contact with her birth father and Joey, but there seems to be no deep attachment on either side: all seem unable to re-connect the emotional cord severed so many years ago. The great benefit in meeting her biological family is that she now knows the full story of her life, and recognizes her close bonds with us. She has no interest in meeting her birth mother, whose drinking, we are told, continues out of control.

Early on October 6, 1997, Brian, Colette and I headed off to see Dr. Brown, whose office in southern Ontario was a long car trip for us. We took an inch-thick file of school reports and psycho-educational assessments, a number of Colette's baby pictures, and the dental moulds of her formerly receding jaw (often seen in people with FAS) supplied by her orthodontist. I had also written a letter summing up the history of our tumultuous relationship with Colette.

Dr. Brown did not look at any of the material I had brought. Colette was looking chic and beautiful, and she told him about her goals: to get off the street, get a job, go back to school, go to college, work with animals. He asked her if she'd ever had a job. Oh, yes, she said, she'd had numerous jobs, and she listed them all. (She neglected to mention she'd turned up for one job for twelve hours; that she'd been fired from another one within three days.) We tried to explain what we had been dealing with—learning difficulties, stealing, bank fraud, addiction—but he didn't seem interested.

Finally, Brian and I spoke bluntly. It was difficult to do in her presence because we didn't want to seem to be blaming her. I said that she often appeared to have no conscience and no ability to learn from experience, and Brian told the doctor a little about our life in the past seven years. We explained that our research indicated that her birth mother's alcohol consumption might explain some of this behaviour. Dr. Brown asked how much her mother had drunk per day during those binges. I said we'd been told that she would be drunk for as long as three weeks at a time. "How many drinks would that take?" he asked. I didn't know. As a non-drinker, how could I know how much booze it would take to keep a woman drunk for that period of time?

Measuring Colette's head size, Dr. Brown found it normal. He said that because of her size (nearly five foot seven and, even after her weight loss, about 150 pounds), she did not seem to be suffering from her mother's alcoholism. But by then we knew from our research that persons with FASD can have normal head size, height and weight. We knew that Colette displayed numerous other symptoms in the FASD constellation—heart murmur, frequent ear problems, slight scoliosis, learning disabilities, insensitivity to pain and temperature, sugar craving, jaw malocclusion, hairy body as a small child, addiction and the seeming lack of conscience. Dr. Brown wrote a prescription for her current ear infection, and sent her off to get some heart tests.

When she returned, he told us it was "normal" for teenagers to rebel, and that she was probably simply going through a "stage." But for nearly four years I had worked as a volunteer with parents of acting-out children, and knew that Colette's behaviour was extreme. If Colette had not been sitting beside me, I would have asked, Is it "normal" for a young woman to spend her fourteenth summer on the street, surviving by panhandling or worse? Is it normal for a fourteen-year-old to put a knife to her sister's throat and threaten to kill her? Is it normal for a seventeen-year-old to constantly steal money and other belongings from her family, to be addicted to crack and to live with a thirty-seven-year-old speed addict in a building described by police as "a hotbed of prostitution"?

Dr. Brown told us Colette was "a very high-functioning person, with a lot of intelligence and insight," and that she was capable of making her own decisions and setting her own goals, and that Brian and I should let go and allow her to do so. "Is she capable of living independently? Isn't that what she is doing right now?" he asked. Yes (we didn't say), except she is living on the street, and it's only a matter of time before she gets arrested for some kind of crime, or before the police find her dead of an overdose.

"Are you saying that the amount of substance her birth mother consumed during pregnancy has not affected Colette's behaviour?" I asked. He said we were possibly "on the right track" but that he didn't want to put a label on Colette's behaviour, as this was "a grey area." He added that he did not want to give her "an excuse" for her behaviour.

We drove home stunned and enraged, while Colette slept in the back seat, looking as angelic as when she was four. We didn't want a label either, just an explanation. If she'd had a rare genetic disease, wouldn't he have told us the truth? A diagnosis was the only way we could stop blaming her and stop blaming ourselves, and seek new directions. The following morning, I wrote a post to my friends at FASlink:

> It would have been helpful if he had read the school reports and said that there was a strong possibility that she wasn't lazy, that she had been doing the best she could, and possibly the schools should have changed their environment so she could have learned better . . .
>
> [Or] if he had said that FAE makes it harder for people to make good judgments, and that somehow we had to work together to figure out a way so that she could stop acting so impulsively. Or if he'd

said that she had spent nine months in an extremely addictive environment, that she must get rehab, and that she must avoid drugs and alcohol as she is extremely vulnerable . . . My sense is that he didn't want to hurt her feelings, but by not being straightforward about this real affliction he didn't help her one bit.

Last night when we got back, Colette's throat was hurting, and as she packed her knapsack, she said, 'I wish I didn't have to go back to the Selby Hotel [the fleabag where she was staying with her then 'boyfriend.']

I said, "I wish you didn't, too.' Then I drove her to the subway, we both cried, I gave her money for subway tickets (most of which will probably go on cigarettes and drugs) and she went off in the night, and I came home.

A few weeks later, she was "in love" again. He was a weird giant with a history of mental illness and incarceration due to violence, and Colette came barely to his shoulder. "Ryan" collected monthly disability benefits, which he always managed to blow within two days. He and Colette were now living in a tent in a Toronto ravine, a few blocks from the downtown core. He told us about his alcoholic parents and how he'd left home at an early age—and I wondered whether he too was a victim of prenatal alcohol. Colette viewed him as her protector, but he seemed to be a mass of barely contained rage, and I feared she would be a victim.

She would be eighteen in January, an adult under Canadian law, and there seemed to be no way we could head off an inevitable disaster. By the time we made the trip to Dr. Brown, I had obsessively researched FASD for seven months. Those countless e-mail messages every day from around three hundred FASlink correspondents confirmed that we all had, more or less, the same child. In my gut, I knew what I was dealing with. But why were the professionals so ignorant of fetal alcohol and so afraid of "labelling"? Brian began to call FASD the "invisible plague." Sick at heart, we took down the childhood photographs of Colette: on horseback, nose to nose with a baby goat at Vancouver's Stanley Park, briefly wearing a dainty pink sundress at age four. It was too heart-breaking to look at these reminders of the days when we naively believed that nurture could conquer nature.

I was still seeing the grief therapist, Lynne. At my first session with her after the failed diagnosis, I tried to deal with the anguish and fear I was feeling about Colette, and my anger at Dr. Brown. Experienced in both addictions and neurological trauma, Lynne was appalled that Dr. Brown had made a diagnosis without doing any neuropsychiatric testing. She assured me that I wasn't wrong to suspect that FASD was the source of Colette's problems. "But, why *is* it so important to you to have a diagnosis?" she asked.

It took me a while to come up with an answer. "Because I have to know there's nothing more I can do."

"Well, you're wrong," said Lynne. "It's possible that more *could* be done." She told me about the work she had been doing in neurological trauma in a large downtown hospital. "I've seen people come in after car accidents—they're unable to walk or talk because of severe brain damage. The situation seems hopeless, but after a program of specialized therapy, they leave walking and talking. It might be possible to map the lesions of the brain of someone with FAS and train other parts of the brain to take over. Just because it's not being done right now for people with fetal alcohol damage doesn't mean it might not be done in the future."

I remembered that two mothers in the state of Washington had tried a series of neurobiofeedback sessions (a kind of brain retraining) on their children with FAS, and had reported a degree of success. Lynne's words encouraged me to keep trying to get a diagnosis, and within the same week, a FASlink friend suggested I get in touch with her colleague Dr. Ab Chudley of Winnipeg, a respected pediatric geneticist and researcher in FAS.

Dr. Chudley responded to my e-mail within twenty-four hours and suggested I send him Colette's file. I photocopied every document we had, including her medical history; adoption records including non-identifying information from CAS; school history and psycho-educational tests; childhood photos; records from Hincks; samples of her schoolwork, letters and a journal. I also wrote a letter detailing what we knew about her parents' substance abuse, plus her own quirks, behaviour, addictiveness and the many wonderful qualities that kept us fighting for her. I enclosed photographs of Colette from the age of ten months to the present. Again, we waited.

By mid-November, when we headed off to the conference on FAS at Ann Arbor, Colette had fallen in love again, this time with "Greg," who had been on the streets for several years. They were bunking in a friend's room in a low-cost residence downtown, operated by the City of Toronto. Almost every resident in the building was on social assistance, and on the first of each month, when the government cheques arrived, everybody partied like crazy for a day or two. Then, having blown their income on drugs, alcohol and junk food, they "worked" as squeegee kids or panhandlers. I suspected that many people in this building were suffering from prenatal alcohol damage: almost all seemed unable to link cause and effect, and were highly addictive and unemployable. Most of them displayed another FASD quality: they were extremely generous, sharing everything with Colette—housing, food, and unfortunately alcohol and drugs.

Colette was not entitled to welfare as she was not yet eighteen; Greg could not get it either, because like most street people he had lost or thrown away all of his identification years earlier. (Not having identification means that you can give the police a phony name or address.) Unskilled school dropouts, both were virtually unemployable. So they had joined the squeegee brigade—standing at the side of busy intersections with a pail of water and a squeegee, running out to wash windshields when the light changed, requesting a dollar or two.

On December 6 I received an e-mail from Dr. Chudley: "I have mailed you my assessment . . . Yes, and unequivocally, your daughter has Alcohol-Related Neurodevelopmental Disorder [ARND, a.k.a. FAE]." A detailed letter arrived a few days later. Like a medical Hercule Poirot, this compassionate man had pored over those thick files. He'd written three single-spaced pages about what he had read, and he seemed to know her as well as we did, without having met her. A diagnosis of ARND, he concluded, was unquestionable. It would be extremely difficult for her to hold a job, handle money or be a responsible parent:

> She needs to live in a protective family-like environment or group home where unlawful acts can be limited and she can be properly supervised. Academics are not her strength and she should be encouraged to learn a vocation. Her self-esteem is low because of the continued failures she has experienced. Unfortunately the school has just not reckoned with the fact that these children have a neurologic condition and their difficulties are not due to laziness or lack of cooperation.

Since 1997 I have encountered numerous adoptive parents who have undergone equally frustrating experiences in their attempts to find answers to their children's puzzling behaviour. Teresa Kellerman of the FAS Family Resource Centre in Tucson, Arizona, says that of the hundreds of letters and e-mails she has received from adoptive parents, two-thirds have figured out that their children have prenatal alcohol damage not through professionals, but through media such as television or magazines.

For many parents, the Aha! moment is followed by a series of barriers. Who in your area can make a definite diagnosis? Numerous psychological tests must be administered and interpreted. A geneticist must rule out any similar disorders caused by genes rather than prenatal alcohol. The diagnostician must know how much alcohol was consumed by the birth mother, and that information is usually nonexistent or unavailable—often sealed in a file if the child is adopted. Even if the biological parents can be tracked down, it may be impossible to confirm maternal drinking in pregnancy. The biological mother may not remember whether she drank, or how much she consumed. Another problem is that few diagnosticians are familiar with the subtle symptoms of central nervous system damage seen in seemingly normal young people with ARND. Unfortunately, "Dr. Brown" was typical of the many physicians who do not keep up with the latest criteria developed at

University of Washington's Department of Medicine, the world's leading specialists in diagnosing fetal alcohol disorders.

For Brian and me, just knowing what we were dealing with helped us enormously. Now we could begin to build a new kind of relationship with Colette. But, unfortunately, there were no resources in Ontario specific to her needs.

Christmas 1997. After six months of living on the street, Colette was fed up with homelessness, parties and drugs, and when she turned eighteen in January, she would be eligible for welfare. She and Greg asked Brian and me to help them get off the street. It took me several weeks of dealing with endless red tape and driving around in snowstorms to get Colette on welfare and help them find a small, clean, affordable apartment, with a landlord who would accept people on social assistance. I also had to help Greg deal with the probation officer he had been avoiding for six months. To pay first and last month's rent for their apartment, we cashed bonds purchased years earlier for Colette's university education years: even a high school diploma for Colette was among those vanished dreams.

On February 1, 1998, an icy, snowy day, Colette and Greg moved into their small apartment, assisted by both Colette's birth father and Brian. We found it ironic that although some of our friends had children who were completing graduate school, we were probably happier than most of them. Our daughter was living on welfare, but we now knew for certain the cause of her lifelong problems. More important, for the first time in many months, we could go to sleep knowing she was safe.

CHAPTER FIVE

The Myth of the Safe Threshold

*We know of no safe time period, we know of no safe [alcoholic]
beverage, and we know of no person who bears a child who
is not vulnerable at some level of drinking. So . . . I must say
that . . . the safest course of action for pregnant women is
abstinence.*

—DR. R. E. LITTLE, A PIONEER RESEARCHER IN FAS

In 1988, while eight-year-old Colette struggled to learn the difference
between b's and d's, the FAS researcher Dr. Kenneth Lyons Jones
showed photos of fifty-four babies to the United States Senate subcommittee that was studying proposed legislation on warning labels
on alcohol beverage containers. He explained that all fifty-four had
been born to women who had consumed only one or two ounces of
absolute alcohol a day during their pregnancies. Yet six of these babies,
born to "moderate" drinkers—eleven percent—had been diagnosed
with fetal alcohol syndrome!

Dr. Jones was one of the authors of the original University of
Washington study that first defined fetal alcohol syndrome; Senator Al
Gore, later the vice-president, was chairing the subcommittee hearings.
According to Congress Hearings records, Dr. Jones then explained to
Senator Gore that between one and two ounces of absolute alcohol is

equivalent to two to four shots of hard liquor, two to four beers or two to four five-ounce glasses of wine:

> We are talking here about a woman who is making dinner that night, and as she does so, she drinks a glass of wine. Her husband comes home and they sit down for dinner, and she has another glass of wine with her husband.

Dr. Jones added that this woman has just consumed an ounce of pure alcohol, and if she is pregnant, she "has an 11 percent chance of having a baby with a prenatal effect of alcohol." Gore, stunned, asked Dr. Jones:

> Now a lot of women who consider themselves in the category of moderate drinkers would come home from work and have a couple of glasses of wine and then maybe during dinner another glass of wine and feel they are in the moderate drinker category. And yet, you are saying that women in that category, if they continue that allegedly moderate drinking during pregnancy . . . have an 11 percent chance that their child, born of that pregnancy, will have the effects of this fetal alcohol syndrome? Is that correct?

Dr. Jones answered, "That is correct. Yes."

Gore stated, "That is really astounding."[12]

Legislation requiring warning labels was passed by the U.S. government shortly after that conversation, and fifteen years later, the United States remains the only country in the world in which all alcohol beverage containers warn against consuming alcohol in pregnancy. But the message of early researchers Little and Jones—that pregnant women who drink occasionally or "moderately" can also harm their babies—has not yet reached the consciousness of many professionals or the general public.

When I first hit FASlink, I sometimes wondered if my worldwide e-mail buddies were suffering from acute paranoia. Living twenty-four hours a day with our children with FASD, most of us knew far more

THE MYTH OF THE SAFE THRESHOLD

about this disorder than the doctors, therapists, teachers, lawyers and judges our kids encountered. Our homes were cluttered with stacks of medical studies and piles of books about FASD, and all of us were aware of two facts:

- Millions of children and adults worldwide are struggling with lost intellectual potential caused by prenatal alcohol, and most will never be diagnosed.
- More than thirty years of research indicates *there is no guaranteed safe threshold of alcohol in pregnancy.*

Why were these messages not getting out?

Nine Deadly Myths about Alcohol in Pregnancy

Some of my activist friends believe they are up against an international conspiracy driven by the alcohol industries, which have managed to co-opt key members of the medical profession, governments and the media, with the result that the message about FASD is not getting out. But is it a conspiracy, a conflict of interest or just ignorance on the part of professionals, caused by information overload? Or can this apathy be traced to the various myths that professionals and the general public mistakenly believe? Here are nine of those myths:

- There is a safe threshold of consumption of alcohol in pregnancy.
- There are safe times in pregnancy when it's okay to drink.
- Only alcoholic women can damage their children by drinking in pregnancy.
- Smoking and street drug use in pregnancy are more dangerous than alcohol.
- There's no point in diagnosing a person with prenatal damage because nothing can be done to help.

- Many women drink throughout pregnancy and their babies are just fine. [This is a dangerous assumption. Although some alcohol-exposed infants do escape injury, others may have learning or behaviour problems that are not apparent until they begin school.]
- Small amounts of wine in pregnancy can help you relax, and are good for baby too.
- People who warn you of the dangers of occasional drinking in pregnancy are evangelical fanatic do-gooders.
- If we warn women who have accidentally consumed alcohol in early pregnancy, they will get anxious, or abort perfectly healthy fetuses.

Is There a Safe Threshold?

Remember that, unlike tobacco, marijuana, cocaine and heroin, alcohol is a "teratogen"—a substance that causes permanent birth defects. Its effects are "dose-dependent," which means that the more a woman consumes in pregnancy, the greater the risk to her baby. Other famous teratogens include thalidomide, codeine and toluene (used in glue-sniffing): would we suggest to a woman that even a "moderate" amount of any of these might be safe?

In 1974 Dr. Ann Streissguth and her team at the University of Washington began examining the long-term effects of "moderate" prenatal alcohol exposure on 486 infants born to mothers who consumed two or more drinks per day (one ounce of absolute alcohol), or consumed five or more drinks on any occasion in the month before learning they were pregnant. These mothers were not considered to be at high risk of producing a child with FAS: all were white, married and middle-class, all received prenatal care by the fifth month of pregnancy. The children were examined after birth; at eight and eighteen months; at four years; at seven; and at seven and a half.

By the age of seven, the children were all of average intelligence.

But researchers found that the youngsters whose mothers had consumed two or more drinks per day had IQs seven points lower than would otherwise have been expected. These children also had learning and behaviour problems in the areas of co-operation, sustained attention, retention of information, comprehension of words, impulsiveness, tact, word recall, and organizational skills. *Children of women who had drunk more than five drinks on any occasion in the month before recognition of pregnancy were generally one to three months behind children of abstainers in reading and arithmetic skills.* Twenty-four percent of the children of "moderate drinkers" were participating in remedial school programs, compared with 15 percent of the children of abstainers.

Six months later—at age seven and a half—the children were given additional tests. The results indicated that low amounts of prenatal alcohol *are* related to attention and memory deficits, as well as distractibility, inflexibility, and poor organizational skills. The performance deficits occurred despite "average" IQs, suggesting central nervous system damage that was too subtle to be picked up by IQ tests.[13]

There's scientific evidence that even *one* episode of binge drinking (defined as four to five drinks over the course of a few hours) in pregnancy can permanently damage the fetus. A team of international researchers at Washington University School of Medicine in St. Louis, Missouri, reported their findings in *Science* magazine in February 2000. Using baby rats going through a spurt of brain growth equivalent to that of a fetus in the third trimester, researchers exposed them, just once, to high concentrations of alcohol for about four hours. This high concentration, a dose equivalent to twice the legal limit for driving in many parts of the world, was found to kill off groups of nerve cells and cause permanent neurological damage. By changing the times at which the baby rats were exposed to alcohol, the researchers triggered nerve-cell loss from many different regions of the brain.[14]

Subtle, Permanent Effects

*Your typical woman in Northern Ireland spontaneously cuts
down on alcohol during pregnancy—but she's told that it's okay
to have a few drinks. I became aware that there really is no safe
level. There were warnings here saying "Don't drink when you're
pregnant. Alcohol can damage your unborn baby"—but there
was just no awareness here at all. I went into my study not
really expecting huge differences—but I did find huge differences
in the startle response and in habituation.*

—Dr. Jennifer Little, a researcher at Queen's
University, Belfast, Northern Ireland

In the summer of 1999 a young psychologist from Belfast, Northern
Ireland, made a presentation at a meeting of the British Psychological
Society. Dr. Jennifer Little's paper generated worldwide media attention.
Newspapers as far away as India and South Africa reported her findings,
which indicated that "moderate" alcohol consumption can cause neurological damage to the fetus. She had studied 128 babies of mothers who
smoke and drank in pregnancy, testing them in the womb at twenty-five
weeks' gestation and following them up as infants. Her research at
Belfast's Royal Maternity Hospital indicated that pregnant women who
drank as little as four units of alcohol per week—equivalent to two pints
of beer or four small glasses of wine—were affecting the wiring of their
infants' brains.[15] Mothers were included in the drinking group if they
reported consuming at least one unit of alcohol (one standard drink)
per week in pregnancy. The mean number of alcohol units consumed
was just over an ounce of pure alcohol per week. "I didn't expect lower
levels of alcohol to have as great an impact on the behaviour of the
fetus," Dr. Little told Trevor McDonald of the British ITV channel. "The
fact that we found those differences in fetuses of mothers who weren't
actually drinking that much alcohol was quite significant."

Dr. Little explained to me that all women who came to the hospital for antenatal (prenatal) care were invited to participate. The women

enjoyed doing it, "because they had more ultrasound scans and more photos than they would have otherwise. They brought their partners and other children, and it was really nice because it turned into a wee family thing."

The tests involved ultrasound monitoring of the fetal response to a "vibroacoustic stimulator" (a kind of buzzer), sometimes used by obstetricians. The fetuses were first tested at twenty-five weeks' gestation, when the startle response usually emerges. They were tested again at thirty-two weeks and thirty-eight weeks, and at five months after birth. The buzzer would be placed against the mother, and the fetus's reaction would be checked. A healthy fetus would respond immediately, extending its limbs, straining its back and turning its head—and then returning to a resting position. Seventy percent of fetuses whose mothers abstained from alcohol responded normally. But among smokers and drinkers, only 32 percent of fetuses responded normally. The results indicated that although together smoking and drinking affected the brain stem, alcohol on its own had a much more profound effect than tobacco.

At the age of five months, all of the infants were tested using slides of female faces, to see how quickly they "habituated" to new information. Again, the infants exposed to any amount of prenatal alcohol habituated less quickly than the infants who had not been exposed prenatally.

Part of Dr. Little's research was published in August 2002 in the British medical journal *Physiology and Behaviour*. The article notes the strong difference in startle response between the five-month fetuses whose mothers abstained and those whose mothers drank any amount at all. No mother had any alcohol in her body during the fetal tests.[16]

"Spontaneous startles" begin at about eight weeks of gestation, and appear as rapid movements beginning in the limbs and spreading through the body. Compared to the fetuses of abstaining mothers, the fetuses exposed to any amount of prenatal alcohol exhibited a significantly higher frequency of spontaneous startles, but 60 percent did not exhibit a startle response to the buzzer. Although these children of occasional drinkers showed no physical signs of fetal alcohol damage at birth, 60 percent had abnormal neurological reactions, which could affect learning and behaviour. Dr. Little told me that these results indicate a direct effect of alcohol on brain-stem functioning, as a fetus needs a fully functioning brain stem to exhibit a startle response. Moreover, she found deviations in neurobehavioural functioning at all gestational ages, abnormalities that continued after birth. She concludes that "the effect of alcohol on the fetus is not transient but permanent."

Dr. Pat Troop, the British government's deputy chief medical officer, was interviewed on the same ITV show that featured Dr. Little, and defended the government's guideline of four units (about four five-ounce glasses of wine) per week. "We could not find evidence that occasional drinking did any harm. We don't want women to feel guilty that if they have an occasional drink it is going to cause a problem."[17] About two-thirds of British women drink in pregnancy. The Royal College of Obstetricians and Gynaecologists recommends "no more than one standard drink per day."[18] Both the British government and the Royal College are ignoring the research indicating that even small amounts of prenatal alcohol can permanently, and subtly, affect an individual's learning and behaviour. Most informed women who are not addicted to alcohol would probably feel that these occasional drinks are just not worth the risk.

Behaviour Problems

At Detroit's Wayne State University, researchers compared seven-year-old children of occasional and moderate drinkers with those whose mothers had abstained, and their findings were reported in the August 2001 issue of *Pediatrics*. The researchers followed a group of children of light or social drinkers from pregnancy to age seven. The families were of African-American heritage, representing the primary clientele of the clinic. Beginning in 1986, women attending the university-based maternity clinic were screened for drug and alcohol use at their first prenatal visit. All women reporting alcohol consumption at conception of at least half an ounce of absolute alcohol per day were invited to help the researchers identify the effects of prenatal alcohol on child development (half an ounce of absolute alcohol is equivalent to the British "unit" of alcohol used by Dr. Little: twelve ounces of beer, five ounces of wine, or one and a half ounces of distilled spirits). Some lower level drinkers and abstainers chosen at random were also invited to participate.

At each prenatal visit, the women were interviewed about alcohol use during the previous two weeks. Alcohol intake was categorized into no alcohol, low intake (less than 0.3 ounces of absolute alcohol per day) and moderate/heavy intake (greater than 0.3 ounces of absolute alcohol per day.) Six years later, 665 families were contacted, and 501 family groups were tested. Almost 25 percent of the women had said they didn't drink in pregnancy. Sixty-four percent reported low levels of use, and 13 percent reported moderate to heavy use. "Increasing prenatal alcohol exposure was associated with lower birth weight and gestational age, lower education level, prenatal exposure to cocaine and smoking, custody changes, lower socioeconomic status, and paternal drinking and drug use at the time of pregnancy," says the report. Various personality tests assessed the children for aggressive and delinquent behaviour, and anxious/depressed and withdrawn behaviour. The researchers found that *children who had encountered any amount of prenatal alcohol had a much higher incidence of both aggressive and delinquent behaviour.* The effect was observed at average levels of exposure of as low as one drink per week, and the researchers concluded:

> Children with any prenatal alcohol exposure were 3.2 times as likely to have Delinquent behavior scores in the clinical range compared with nonexposed children. The relationship between prenatal alcohol exposure and adverse childhood behavior outcome persisted after controlling for other factors associated with adverse behavioral outcomes. Clinicians are often asked by pregnant women if small amounts of alcohol intake are acceptable during pregnancy. These data suggest that no alcohol during pregnancy remains the best medical advice.

After spending every Thursday night for five years supporting countless desperate parents of delinquent teenagers, I now believe that many of those youngsters may have struggled lifelong with invisible brain damage caused by "moderate" amounts of prenatal alcohol. Most had normal or above-normal intelligence, and the majority had been diagnosed with attention deficit hyperactivity disorder. Those devoted middle-class mothers in my support group would never have been considered alcoholics, but many of them looked forward to their daily glasses of wine, before and during dinner. If no doctor had warned them that this moderate drinking could affect their unborn child, they would have had no reason to stop.

Why Doctors Don't Know

Our results show that many [obstetrical] textbooks, even recently, seem to have interpreted the absence of a "safe level" to mean that lower amounts of alcohol are safe and may be permitted. However, alcohol rapidly moves to the fetal circulation and is toxic to fetal cells . . . Inconsistent recommendations are not appropriate because they leave the reader with the impression that abstinence is the official line but a foolish rule made to be broken.

—Karen Q. Loop and Mary D. Nettleman, M.D.,
"Obstetrical Textbooks: Recommendations about
Drinking during Pregnancy," American Journal of
Preventive Medicine (August 2002)

Many women who became mothers in recent years have told me that when they were pregnant their doctors failed to ask them about alcohol consumption. Several others have said that their doctors told them that small amounts of alcohol were not harmful, and could even be beneficial.

In 2000 researchers Karen Loop and Dr. Mary Nettleman of Virginia Commonwealth University began reviewing current textbooks in obstetrics, looking at information regarding alcohol in pregnancy. Searching eighty-one texts, they were surprised that only fourteen (17 percent) contained a consistent recommendation that pregnant women should not drink alcohol. Their article, cited above, indicates that more than half of obstetrical texts had at least one statement condoning drinking in pregnancy; 24 percent contained a discussion without recommendations; and 6 percent were silent.

They add that twenty-nine books gave inconsistent recommendations—often one section would recommend abstinence, while another would state that lower amounts were safe. In two cases, they found inconsistency in a single sentence, such as "abstinence is recommended but one drink a day is probably permissible." (The Belfast psychologist Dr. Jennifer Little found that one drink a day was unlikely to cause FAS, but could result in permanent effects in learning and reaction to stimulus.) Loop and Nettleman were dismayed that of the twenty texts published since 1991, only seven consistently recommended abstinence.

Misleading Manuals

Intrigued by the research of Loop and Nettleman, I began looking at recent manuals published for pregnant women. Examining the most popular books on Amazon, at a large book chain and in the public library, I found that most authors stressed the potential damage of tobacco, prescription drugs and street drugs, but suggested that light or occasional drinking is harmless. Several authors advised women who had binge-drunk before realizing they were pregnant not to worry, telling them that it was unlikely they had damaged their babies. They cited stories of women who had been worried, but then gave birth to "perfectly healthy" infants. These authors seem unaware that fetal alcohol damage is often invisible—that the child's subtle neurological problems may not emerge until he or she hits school, worsening in adolescence.

Vicki Iovine, author of the number one best-seller, *The Girlfriends' Guide to Pregnancy: Or Everything Your Doctor Won't Tell You,* is the worst offender. She rants about the "Pregnancy Police" who lecture pregnant women who have a glass of wine with dinner—and suggests that "women coming to the end of a healthy and uneventful pregnancy" should soothe their insomnia with a glass of wine or a hot toddy. Several other books suggest that women avoid alcohol during the first trimester when fetal organs are forming—and after that allow themselves one or two drinks per week. The research of the Wayne State team and Belfast's Dr. Jennifer Little indicates that this amount could permanently affect the child's learning and behaviour. Among books giving risky advice are *Pregnancy for Dummies,* written by Joanne Stern, M.D., and Keith Eddleman, M.D., faculty members of Mount Sinai Hospital in New York City, and journalist Mary Murray; and *The Everything Pregnancy Book,* by Maryann Brinley and Howard Berk, M.D.

The Complete Book of Pregnancy and Childbirth, by the respected British childbirth educator Sheila Kitzinger, originally published in 1980, has been revised several times, most recently in 2000, but does not look at recent research on alcohol. Kitzinger writes, "Most women can drink in moderation in pregnancy and have a perfect baby. Limit your alcohol to ten units per week and do spread them out over the week." Ten units a week is five ounces of pure alcohol—twice the mean amount studied by Dr. Jennifer Little, which was shown to affect startle and habituation. (One of the key characteristics of FASD noted by Dr. Ann Streissguth is "difficulty modulating incoming stimuli: poor habituation.")[19] The book's cover indicates that more than a million copies have been sold.

None of these authors seem aware of the studies indicating that beautiful, physically healthy babies may nevertheless have invisible central nervous system damage caused by prenatal alcohol—damage that can cause permanent attention deficits, aggression and learning problems. Like codeine, alcohol is a teratogen. It causes birth defects. I wonder how many mothers who have followed the above authors' advice have found themselves dealing with children struggling with puzzling learning disabilities and attention deficit disorders. I also question whether these "experts" would suggest that a pregnant woman take a codeine-laced painkiller, on the grounds that risk to the fetus is slight.

I found only three current pregnancy guides that recognize the dangers of "moderate" drinking. *What to Expect When You're Expecting*, by Arlene Eisenberg, Heidi E. Murkoff and Sandee E. Hathaway, describes both FAS and FAE, and says, "The safe daily alcohol dose in pregnancy, if there is one, is not known." Canadian author Ann Douglas's *The Mother of All Pregnancy Books* repeatedly advises "no alcohol" and suggests that hubby abstain as well. However, both of these books suggest that the occasional drink probably won't hurt baby.

The Pregnancy Book for Today's Woman by Howard Shapiro, M.D., earns my A+ for Accuracy. In the only manual I found that thoroughly covers recent research on prenatal alcohol, Shapiro writes:

> Minimal alcohol consumption during pregnancy should not be condoned, since susceptibility varies from one woman to another, and since subtle anatomic and neurological defects in newborns are often not detected until late in childhood.

Misinformed Media

If pregnant women journalists are getting incorrect information in the manuals they read, is it any wonder that the media are sending the message that so-called "light" or "moderate" drinking is harmless?

In early 2003, on a local radio show with an audience of several hundred thousand, a female announcer cracked open a bottle of champagne, on air, to share with an eight-months pregnant female technician who was going on maternity leave. "It's safe now," the announcer said, pouring bubbly for her pregnant colleague. When I wrote to the producer, pointing out that no amount of alcohol in pregnancy can ever be guaranteed to be safe, the announcer defensively wrote back: "Most medical experts concede that the total abstinence doctrines of caffeine, tobacco and alcohol consumption are the rule only because some pregnant women are incapable of extreme moderation. We don't need to infantilize [our] educated and mature listeners." The "educated and mature" announcer, herself a recent mother, is obviously unaware that unlike caffeine and tobacco, alcohol is a teratogen that can cause defects in the developing fetus.

A few weeks later, I was interviewed about FASD on an educational TV show. The story researcher had requested documentation, so I'd sent abstracts of numerous medical research studies. Even so, the female host could not believe the research, and asked me, almost angrily, during the interview: "Well, what *are* small amounts of alcohol? My small amount might not be the same as someone else's small amounts!" I told her about the University of Washington and Wayne State University research: children whose mothers have consumed *any* alcohol at all in pregnancy have a higher risk of learning problems, attention deficits and aggressive behaviour than children of mothers who abstained. She shook her head, as if I were making it up.

Warning Labels

Failure to label alcohol beverages when medical drugs, foods, cleaners, solvents and other dangerous products all carry health warnings falsely assures consumers that alcoholic beverages are safe at all times.

—PAUL SZABO, M.P., THE REAL BRAIN DRAIN

Legislation was enacted in the United States in 1988 requiring alcohol beverage containers to have labels warning against alcohol consumption in pregnancy, when driving a car or when using heavy machinery. Eight other countries (Brazil, Colombia, Costa Rica, Ecuador, Honduras, Mexico, South Korea and Zimbabwe) have mandated warning labels on alcohol beverage containers, but they warn only of health problems such as cirrhosis and/or the dangers of drinking if driving or operating heavy machinery. Despite work by advocates in Canada, Great Britain, Australia and New Zealand, the U.S. remains the only country in which alcoholic beverage containers must indicate that consumption in pregnancy can permanently hurt the fetus. As this book goes to press, however, the South African government has indicated it will legislate mandatory warning labels on alcoholic beverage containers.

In 1995, in Canada, a private members bill on labelling was put forward in the House of Commons by Paul Szabo, Liberal Member of Parliament for Mississauga South (adjacent to Toronto). Szabo's bill died when the House of Commons subcommittee on health voted to delay it, knowing it would die when the next election was called. Szabo maintains that the bill was sabotaged by the alcohol industry, which had mounted an aggressive $100,000 lobbying campaign. He also says that the Brewers Association of Canada (now called Brewers of Canada) threatened to cancel $10 million in funding to the government-sponsored Canadian Centre on Substance Abuse (CCSA).

Nearly a decade later, two more private members' bills on this issue have been proposed and nothing has been done. Szabo, who spent many years as a senior corporate accountant, says of the alcohol beverage industry:

> I've often thought they will graciously support programs that they feel are generally neutral in terms of impact on their business. But as soon as you get close to the bone, and you start talking about things that may very well work, then you get the reaction . . . "if you legislate warning labels, then we will withdraw funding in other areas." (Interview with author)

Could part of the problem encountered by Paul Szabo and international activists be the fact that alcohol is big business everywhere? In Canada, the combined tax revenues from the alcohol industry, provincially and federally, are $3.2 billion per year. The U.S. alcohol industry adds $65 billion a year to the American economy, including about two billion per year on advertising and promotion. Few media can afford to ignore these valuable corporate revenues.

In addition, U.S. breweries sponsor about 10 percent of all athletic, musical and cultural events—and promote their wares at sports events, rock concerts and college "spring break" activities that generally attract large audiences of underage drinkers. In the United States, Canada, the United Kingdom and Australia, consumption of wine and beer is marketed as being associated with financial success and romance, and heavy drinking is seen as a "fun" activity, where no one ever gets drunk, sick, belligerent or accidentally pregnant.

Research by the behavioural scientist Thomas Greenfield and others indicates that the U.S. warning labels have had the effect of slightly reducing alcohol consumption in pregnancy, but that they need to be backed up by other promotional material. The U.S. labels are small, and design and copy have not changed since 1989. Greenfield suggests that any country considering warning labels should rotate labels from the outset, and that introducing new messages to keep them "fresh" would make them more effective.[20]

In Australia, in 1996, the National Food Authority received a request from the National Council of Women to include warnings on labels of alcoholic beverages, indicating the risk of birth defects from prenatal alcohol. Sue Miers of Australia's National Organization for Fetal Alcohol Syndrome and Related Disorders submitted a document citing U.S. research studies that indicate that even "moderate" drinking can be harmful to the fetus. Two women's health researchers, Ilse O'Ferrall and Andrea Shoebridge, countered with their own report, suggesting that labelling can have "a potentially adverse social outcome that has led to unwarranted criticism and victimisation of pregnant women":

> Given the absence of scientific evidence to the contrary, a woman should be able to make her own decisions about her alcohol intake and not be subjected to harassment by perhaps well-meaning but misinformed people . . . Women of child-bearing age may be advised to abstain from alcohol if they intend to become pregnant or as soon as they learn that they are pregnant. Women, however, should also know that an occasional drink during pregnancy or a pattern of having consumed 1–2 drinks a day prior to becoming aware of pregnancy is unlikely to be associated with severe damage to the fetus.

(Ilse O'Ferrall and Andrea Shoebridge, *Women, FAS and Alcoholic Beverage Labelling*)

The O'Ferrall/Shoebridge paper was accompanied by a lengthy bibliography, almost all of it Australian. No references were made to the extensive U.S. research indicating that although moderate drinking will probably not result in any noticeable defects in the infant or toddler, it may cause invisible, undetectable neurological damage that will wreak havoc on the family in later years. The authors based their paper on a study by Dr. I. M. Walpole and associates at Princess Margaret Hospital in Perth, Western Australia, published in 1990.

The Walpole Papers

Over a three-year period, Walpole and his team assessed 605 newborn infants, whose mothers drank varying amounts of alcohol in pregnancy; many of them had also smoked. Twenty-four percent of the women (about 125) were abstainers; 50 percent (300) drank less than one drink daily; 12 percent (about 50) drank one to two drinks daily; 5 percent (30) drank two to three drinks daily; 4 percent (24) drank four drinks daily; and about 4 percent (24) drank more than four drinks per day. Shortly after the infants were born, the researchers measured head circumference, length and weight of infants. They also checked Apgar tests, which measure heart rate, respiratory effort, muscle tone, response to stimulation and skin colour: a perfect score is 10. In the three published studies, researchers found "no significant relationship between low to moderate maternal alcohol intake and fetal outcome."[21]

Newborn Colette, weight 2,970 grams (six pounds, nine ounces) with an Apgar of 9, would have passed the Walpole test with flying colours. "You were a healthy baby," says a document from Toronto's Children's Aid Society. It mentions a heart murmur that "would right itself in time." (She still has the heart murmur, and also has mild scoliosis, diagnosed at age four—both of these are birth defects often found in alcohol-affected children.) When this study was done, in the late 1980s, the Walpole researchers seem to have been unaware that many alcohol-affected children seem perfectly normal at birth. Since that time, however, researchers in FASD have repeatedly stated that *the key symptom of fetal alcohol damage is a damaged central nervous system that affects behaviour and learning*—problems which often do not become evident until the child hits school.

I tracked down the three Walpole reports and sent copies to four North American medical professionals, highly experienced in both research and diagnosis. All four bluntly condemned both the methodology and conclusions and pointed out that the researchers seemed to have no knowledge of the subtle effects of FAE/ARND. They all suggested that the infants should have been followed up for several years. Dr. Gideon Koren, of Toronto's Hospital for Sick Children, wrote:

> The Walpole Study of 1990 cannot be used in any way or shape to show the "safety" of alcohol. It measures outcome at birth. These measures do not predict any of the brain effects of alcohol seen later in FAS-ARND.

Dr. Robert J. Clayton, a geneticist in San Antonio, Texas, who has specialized in FASD, wrote that these studies would not be accepted by peer reviewers today:

> The reason they give for not pushing for abstinence is that it "may have the effect of inducing or promoting guilt and suffering in a group of light or social drinking mothers, particularly when there has been a poor pregnancy outcome." I, as a geneticist, would be able to be more helpful in handling dozens of mothers with that guilt than I currently am able to deal with one child with alcohol related spectrum disorder.

Dr. Ab Chudley, the pediatric geneticist at the University of Manitoba who heads Winnipeg's Clinic for Alcohol and Drug Exposed

Children (CADEC), spoke to me at length on the phone about this "crude" study. He said using an Apgar to assess for FASD was like looking at a newborn's hair and eyes to try to determine what his or her colouring would be at age twelve. "It's a very gross estimate that 'Yes, all four limbs are moving, yes, the baby responds to auditory stimuli.'"

Dr. Jo Nanson, a Saskatchewan neuropsychologist who has been involved in identifying children with FASD for several decades, sent me a thoughtful, detailed critique, explaining that Ann Streissguth's longitudinal studies had used far more sophisticated testing on alcohol-exposed infants: "Things like the infant's alertness and its capacity to soothe itself":

> What is most significant about Streissguth's studies is that the dose-dependent effects of alcohol have persisted over time and become more marked as the children matured and were expected to perform more complex tasks, such as reading and getting along with others.

Walpole's dangerous and misleading information continues to be cited as a reason to not inform the general public about the dangers to the fetus of drinking in pregnancy. For example, in 1996, it was used as a reference by the Brewers Association of Canada, to back up their opposition to warning labels.[22]

Citing the Walpole research, the Department of Neonatal Medicine Protocol Book produced by the state of New South Wales, Australia, states: "Population-based studies have cast doubt on the relationship between light alcohol consumption during pregnancy and subsequent abnormal neurodevelopment in the infant."[23] The Walpole papers formed the basis of the 1998 guidelines of the Royal New Zealand College of Obstetricians and Gynecologists, which indicated that up to fifteen alcoholic drinks per week are safe for the fetus. The organization ignored a well-written presentation by Christine Rogan, then executive director of Fetal Alcohol New Zealand Trust, and the advice of a highly respected international team of FAS researchers—Consuelo Guerri of Spain, Kerstin Stromland of Sweden and Edward Riley of the U.S.—

whose advice had been requested. "There are considerable data that suggest that even low levels of ethanol consumption may be harmful to the fetus," they wrote, concluding that, "While one might advise the pregnant woman who has been drinking less than two units per day that the risk to the fetus is relatively small, it would be clinically prudent to advise abstention during pregnancy."[24]

With Friends Like These, Who Needs Enemies?

The Australian medical profession is up to its stethoscopes in grapes and wine, not only as consumers but also as prescribers and producers. So far, over 160 doctors in Australia have established vineyards. So we have got the largest companies, Lindemans, Penfolds and Hardy's, they are Australia's three largest wine companies and all founded by doctors . . . and about 60 percent of Australia's crush each vintage is processed by vineyards founded by doctors.

—Dr. Philip Norrie, speaking to the "Circle of Wine Writers," London, England

The strong link between the Australian wine industry and the medical profession goes back to 1818, when Dr. William Redfern established a vineyard outside Sydney that exists to this day. Numerous other doctors followed, and began promoting wine as a health beverage, which wine industries worldwide continue to do. Unfortunately, doctor-winemakers outside the U.S. have not been forced by law to place labels on their bottles warning consumers that wine stops being a health beverage in pregnancy. Even worse, an international association of wine-making doctors, called the "Medical Friends of Wine," actively denies that "moderate" drinking can be dangerous to the fetus, citing the flawed Walpole "study" as evidence, despite countless research studies that indicate otherwise. Among them is Dr. David N. Whitten, a California physician and winery owner, who has written a widely distributed

THE MYTH OF THE SAFE THRESHOLD

book, *To Your Health,* which recommends up to eight ounces (250 mL) per day in pregnancy. He goes so far as to say that "Some physicians believe that low doses of alcohol may actually improve the probability for healthy babies and healthy offspring."[25]

Dr. Whitten might change his mind if he met Mercedes Alejandro of Houston, Texas, who wishes she had been better informed, "not only about the dangers of alcohol drinking, but that any amount of alcohol, any time in pregnancy, could make a difference." Mercedes had two episodes of social drinking before she knew she was pregnant. Her son was born in 1982 with microcephaly (small head), developmental delays, hypotonia (poor muscle tone), and partial absence of the corpus callosum, which links the right and left hemispheres of the brain. He did not walk or talk until age three, and had to be taught to crawl. At thirteen, he was diagnosed with Fetal Alcohol Effects.

"I don't remember knowing that I was pregnant for the first two months," Mercedes recalls. "Once I found out, I took good care of myself. It never occurred to me to stop and think, 'Oh, what have I done in the past two months?' and review that, because I was just so excited."

> There are many women like me, who would stop drinking entirely if they thought there was a possibility that they could be pregnant, and they knew that alcohol would put their baby at risk. My son is now an adult, and still many women are not being adequately informed. Although some doctors may tell you that "a glass of wine won't hurt your baby," I would rather err on the side of caution and not drink at all—not take that chance.

CHAPTER SIX

Society's Children

The angels all were singing out of tune
And hoarse with having little else to do,
Excepting to wind up the sun and moon,
Or curb a runaway young star or two . . .
—George Gordon, Lord Byron, "Vision of Judgment"

During the summer and fall of 1997 you could not drive in downtown Toronto without being accosted by a strange-looking individual with tattoos, pierced nose, pierced eyebrows, lips and tongue, who brandished a squeegee and pail of dirty water, wanting to clean your windshield. In my searches for Colette, I had met several of her squeegee friends—all school dropouts whose backgrounds included learning problems, addictions and alcoholic parents. I wondered how many of these young people were also struggling with invisible, undiagnosed FASD.

As professional communicators, Brian and I wondered why the effects of fetal alcohol had been so rarely covered in the press. Ann Streissguth's secondary disabilities study indicated that more than half of all people with FASD were likely to be among the homeless, addicts, the mentally ill and those involved with crime or living on welfare. These people cost taxpayers a fortune in social and medical services and the administration of criminal justice. The public, politicians, professionals and media seemed as unaware as we had been. As a journalist, I had unwittingly stumbled on the story of a lifetime: *an invisible, preventable epidemic that had permanently damaged the brains of countless infants worldwide.* Wondering how many more parents of adoptive children had endured a similar struggle, I asked Colette's permission to write our story. Amazingly, she agreed.

Stevie Cameron, then the editor of the Canadian women's magazine *Elm Street,* assigned me to write a feature. The article, "Society's Child," flew out of my computer in less than three days. Although I had written frankly about our family's problems, Colette requested only two small changes of fact, not to protect herself but because I had got them wrong. "Go ahead, Mom. It's okay with me." As always, I was amazed by her courage and generosity of spirit.

The magazine's photographer, Greg Patek, went with Colette and her boyfriend Greg to their former district one cold Saturday and took some shots of them with squeegees and buckets. His photos were published along with the article in the May 1998 issue; the gritty black-and-white layout showed Colette and Greg cleaning windshields, and there was a stunning full-page portrait of Colette looking bleak and abandoned. Within twenty-four hours, the e-mails and letters began to pour in, mostly from desperate adoptive parents across the country.

The first e-mail I received was from Carol Ramsay, the wife of Jean-françois (J.-f.) Lepage, one of the two courageous young men with FAE who had been interviewed on CBC-TV fourteen months earlier—changing our lives forever. Carol, twenty years older than Jean-françois, had also been interviewed on the program, and I'd been captivated by her keen intelligence, compassion and humour. She wrote:

> My biggest struggle has been in learning how to control my behaviour so as not to make a bad situation worse. I have changed my expectations of our relationship and of him and have taken the pressure off myself to have a marriage just like everyone else's. My second biggest struggle has been in the education of those around me.

The prison system is still very much in the dark. J.-f.'s prison files point to FAS, over and over again. [For example:] "In interview he presents as average in intelligence but extremely immature in his social skills. He has no insight, his judgment is poor and his motivation for treatment is questionable." . . . "There are many unresolved concerns in this case, notably his lack of insight into his criminal actions and inappropriate behaviour." . . . "Remorse is considered to be absent." (All classic and permanent disabilities related to FASD.)

The most difficult thing about FAS is how unpredictable J.f.'s actions are. . . . During the times of great difficulty I reflect on the good times, on the love he openly displays . . . During the bad times, I cry and curse and promise I will seek a divorce. Life with J.-f. is a roller coaster of emotions that will never end.

Despite Carol's determination, in late 2000 her marriage ended. Exhausted from the "roller-coaster" ride, which so many parents of people with FASD describe, she continues to volunteer on behalf of adult offenders struggling with prenatal alcohol damage.

Other letters, mostly from adoptive parents, told of children with rages, unable to learn; runaways, addicted teenagers, daughters who had become "exotic dancers" (an upscale term for strippers and prostitutes), sons languishing in prison. Eva Kuper of Montreal, the adoptive mother of a young man with frequent legal problems, wrote of being in a courtroom when the adoptive son of cabinet minister Jean Chrétien, later prime minister of Canada, was also sent to prison: she had seen the pain on the faces of the young man's parents and marvelled at their constant love and support. None of these correspondents had been told by adoption agencies whether their children's mothers had consumed alcohol in pregnancy, or warned of the possible results if they had. "You get more information from the SPCA when adopting a pet than we were given with our child!" wrote a mother whose young adult son has frequently considered suicide.

The children's behaviour seemed to break into two patterns. Some were like Colette—bright and cooperative until they hit school, when problems began to erupt. Others caused trouble from infancy. Cheryl in Western Canada wrote of a daughter who had drawn younger children into prostitution and drug use:

> She rejected compliments from children at school, choosing to chase them with nails and sharp objects when they dared to play with her chosen friend for the day, and when she was rejected she bent their fingers backward and often cuffed the boys in the head so hard they cried . . .

Like Brian and me, the correspondents had been told that constant, unconditional love would enable them to raise an emotionally healthy child. They too had consulted countless child psychologists and psychiatrists, who admonished them to improve their parenting skills. If the parents seemed relatively well-balanced and normal, they were told that the dysfunctional child was bearing the burden of hidden anger in the family. As we had been, one couple were urged to fight in front of the children—and they too failed in their assignment: fighting was just not part of their pattern of behaviour.

Few of the children had been assessed for fetal alcohol damage. Instead, the professionals chose from a grab-bag of other disorders that, unlike FASD, were in the fourth edition of the *Diagnostic and Statistical Manual of Mental Disorders,* known as DSM-IV. The most frequently diagnosed were reactive attachment disorder, attention deficit hyperactivity disorder, oppositional defiant disorder and conduct disorder. The parents described report cards similar to Colette's— particularly the words "should pay more attention," and "could do better." If the children did well in a small special-education class, they would be put back into the regular classroom: it was as if they had learned to walk well on crutches, so the crutches would be cruelly taken away. Almost all of these children had dropped out of school by the age of fourteen. No wonder: as schoolwork becomes increasingly abstract, children with FASD—who learn in a concrete way—find academic subjects almost impossible to handle.

Virtually every parent wrote about a child who, like Colette, had begun abusing tobacco, marijuana and alcohol at an early age. None of us had realized that, as these substances had been part of our children's prenatal environment, they were biologically predetermined to "self-medicate" to feel normal. A Calgary woman wrote of her son, then twelve, who had "climbed onto the roof through his bedroom window and threatened to jump after being caught with beer at school." Her letter reminded me of Colette, suspended from school at around the same age for pilfering—and sharing—small bottles of alcohol Brian had saved from various air trips. She later told me that from an early age she had drunk all of our family's cough syrup—not even realizing it contained alcohol—just because she liked the taste. In our busy, disorganized household, I never noticed how quickly we seemed to use it up.

Attempting to raise these children had bankrupted these parents financially and emotionally. Misha, a young woman from northern British Columbia, whose family had fostered numerous foster children with FASD, wrote that her parents "eventually gave up fostering because of the sheer hopelessness of it. When we began, we naively thought that all the kids needed was someone to love them, but we were wrong . . . Instead, our family nearly fell apart under the incredible strain these kids brought to our household."

Most adoptive parents had invested retirement savings in psychologists, tutoring and special education; most mothers had been unable to work full time because of their children's problems. The parents wrote of broken marriages and mental breakdowns, of being forced to break off connections with their children to protect themselves and other members of their family. Others were now raising their adopted children's children, and watching the same behaviours emerge in their grandchildren: one couple wrote of twin daughters, now in their thirties, who between them had given birth to twelve alcohol-affected children, all by different fathers.

In almost every letter there was fury at the series of professionals they had visited—nearly all of whom had blamed the parents and failed to zero in on the real reason for their children's difficulties in learning and extreme acting-out behaviour. Marisa, a teacher, wrote of her fifteen-year-old daughter, who had been adopted at age two:

> After reading your article I too got on the Internet, went to the library and started reading everything I could on the subject. Each additional fact was like a bomb going off inside me—because so many things were so suddenly crystal clear. I went into a period of mourning, both for my daughter and for ourselves as parents, and also experienced deep grief over the mistakes we had made out of our ignorance. When I went to the doctor who has been treating my daughter, he didn't even want to see the stuff I had copied from the Net because, he said, 'The causes don't matter; I am just treating the symptoms.'

Despite their children's antisocial behaviour, the parents who wrote me loved them. Like Brian and me, they often caught glimpses of the individual who might have been. Many congratulated Colette for her courage in coming forward. She was living on social assistance and was unlikely to finish high school—but they envied me because my marriage was intact, we had a good relationship with Colette, and she seemed to be no longer in danger.

I received more than a hundred letters from parents alone, from as far away as Austria. They viewed me as the first person they had heard of who might have an answer to the puzzle of their children's learning problems and impossible behaviour. Unlike the professionals, I wasn't going to blame *them*. And unlike their friends and relatives, I would not tell them they were insane to continue loving a dysfunctional child who seemed to have no conscience, no remorse, no loyalty. I had no answers, and in many cases could not direct them to a doctor who could make a diagnosis—even if their children had agreed to it. But I tried to answer each letter personally, because I wanted them to know there was one person in the world who could tell them, "I know what you've endured. I share your pain."

Crash-Test Families

I miss him. The brother who never stopped his temper tantrums when he was younger . . . who destroyed things, lied and stole constantly. I loved him, the brother who is a year younger than I. His teachers complained that he bullied other students, made friends with the bad crowds—and he never seemed to stop doing terrible things even after mom and dad disciplined him over and over. When I reached the age when young people are sensitive about their image, I was outraged when I realized that the things he was doing could possibly have an impact on what other people thought of me. I soon became completely ashamed of him.

—SARAH PAY, EIGHTEEN YEARS OLD

Eighty percent of the individuals with FASD interviewed for Ann Streissguth's secondary disabilities study were raised by adoptive or foster families, or other family members besides their parents. Living in an FASD family is like being a real-life crash-test dummy. The entire family is belted into a car without a steering wheel. Then we're sent zinging down the FAS lane, on an expressway without lines or signs, hurtling over the speed limit and out of control, denting fenders on either side, sometimes crashing over the median, hitting other cars or smashing into a concrete wall. We stumble out of the accident, but before we can pull ourselves together we are belted into the car again and sent off on yet another scary trip driven by an unseen, sinister force.

The FASD crash dummies who do best are those who have been given manuals, steering wheels and a well-marked road with clear signs. Unfortunately, this is rarely the case. Whether the alcohol-affected individual came to the family by birth, adoption or as a foster child, she is unlikely to be diagnosed, particularly if, like about 80 percent of individuals with FASD, she has no obvious mental disabilities or physical characteristics. Even if these are identified, she and her parents are unlikely to get the support they need.

When "crash-test families" are not supported, every citizen suffers. Your fenders get crumpled by our out-of-control youngsters as they careen through life. Your children may be bullied in the schoolyard by bigger kids who have been "kept back"—frustrated children with seemingly no conscience. (My shy, fragile older daughter, Cleo, was terrorized by numerous bullies in her school career: in retrospect, many had learning and behaviour problems, and family histories consistent with FASD.) While innocently going about your day, you may find yourself the victims of road rage or burglary, or worse.

But what happens to the unsupported crash-test families is even more tragic. By the early teens, the affected child may become impossible to live with. The shame that Sarah Pay expresses seems to be classic among both parents and siblings. Generally, one parent—most often the mother—is swallowed up by the needs of the alcohol-affected child. She must deal with phone calls from neighbours, the school and, in some cases, the police. Searching for answers to her child's behaviour, she may spend her life on the phone, or driving the child to appointments with therapists and counsellors. Friends, grandparents and in-laws echo therapists' comments that she is "enabling" the affected child. Family gatherings may become impossible because of this child's behaviour. Siblings may suffer from anxiety or depression. Marriage break-ups are not unusual. By the time the affected child has reached his teens, the situation may have become so desperate that he can no longer live at home. Many of our children will end up on the streets—as Colette did.

Brian and I were luckier than other parents we know—some of whose children vanished forever, or died tragically. Nancy Freeman, who lives in the American Midwest, will grieve forever for her beautiful, beloved young adult daughter Marcie, who died in 1999 of an unintentional overdose of street drugs combined with alcohol:

These kids are such innocents, unable to figure out how to stay out of trouble. Marcie was not a victimizer—instead, she was victimized by being soaked in alcohol prenatally. Then, society delivered its blows—not enough understanding, too much exposure to booze and drugs when she was barely a teenager. And the role of men: as she was in a fallen state, anyone could use her. Naturally, she would also use the people around her, for car rides, food, cash, company, advice, a place to stay for a while.

As family stress increases, the impact on parents and siblings rebounds onto the child with FASD. Angry or just plain exhausted, parents and siblings can't help but treat her differently. Some families try to pretend she is not the reason for family breakdown, but despite her disabilities and often tough exterior, she intuitively knows that she is to blame, and this becomes yet another blow to her fragile self-esteem.

When the family breaks down, the alcohol-affected child suffers the most, because she is the least resilient member of all. Because most money allocated for FASD goes to government institutions and for medical and academic research, the families of the world are bearing the financial and emotional burdens of raising children living with prenatal alcohol damage. Lacking accurate diagnosis, educational facilities for their affected youngsters, resources and respite, FASD families are crumbling from the stress, and so are the majority of alcohol-affected adolescents. Some of these youngsters will be drawn to addiction and crime; others will simply struggle day after day, year after year, wishing their lives could be different, not knowing why just surviving is so difficult.

When in Doubt, Blame the Parents

While researching this book, I asked my many parent correspondents which were the least informed statements they had ever had from a professional. Several people complained of uninformed doctors or therapists who explained their children's learning and behaviour problems by saying, "This is only a phase," or "He will grow out of it."

When I think back to raising Colette, what was hardest was not Colette's difficult behaviour, but the uninformed arrogance and denial of many professionals who shifted the blame to us.

Ottawa's Elspeth Ross still feels burned by the treatment of several professionals when her sons were younger. "What hurt me most were the times when the system blamed me directly." She tells of the time when her younger son was in residential treatment in a psychiatric facility because she and her husband Chris were having great difficulty coping with his acting-out behaviour:

> The psychiatrist said that I was an "over-involved mother" and that our family was wrong for this child—that he actually shouldn't be in our family . . . They wrote into his records that our family was dysfunctional and that I was the cause of the child's problems. The doctor said our son would be better off without a family. When I asked what kind of placement she'd suggest, she said they had nothing to offer.

Elspeth notes that this ignorance still continues—that recently another mother of a seven-year-old girl with FASD received exactly the same treatment from the same facility.

Strategies for Survival

These tragic stories don't have to happen. With diagnosis before the age of six, and an informed family working with schools, professionals and the community, much can be done to reduce those secondary disabilities that cause families and society so much energy, grief and money. At the back of this book, you'll find suggestions for books and websites that outline strategies—and here are some key thoughts from people on the front lines:

The Paradigm Shift

Diane Malbin, the biological mother of an adult child with FASD, has a master's degree in social work and has spent years working with affected children and their families. Brian and I sat in a packed keynote workshop at a conference in Grand Rapids, Michigan, where she enthralled us with ideas for change. *"Don't try harder, try differently,"* she said, explaining the necessity for a "paradigm shift" in attitude. She contrasted the help offered to severely physically disabled children—"Give them a wheelchair"—with our treatment of our cognitively disabled children with FASD: we try to coerce them into changing their behaviours. "But what if the behaviour is the symptom of a physical disability?" she asked. Her concept of the paradigm shift, then, is to change our thinking from "She will not . . ." to "She *can* not . . ."

"What if this child just doesn't get it, can't make connections, can't weigh and evaluate? And what if it's not because he's just being lazy? Or wilful? Or ridiculous? What if it's because he has a physical disability?" Malbin spoke of the need to modify our alcohol-affected children's environment, just as we would change the environment of a child with visual impairment or physical disabilities. I thought back to our home, filled with books, art, plants, memorabilia and *stuff*—which I had always thought of as a "stimulating" environment. Now I know that Colette's mind couldn't cope with the clutter, particularly in her own large, jam-packed room. A small, simple room with only a few toys, books and articles of clothing would have been easier for all of us. And the series of classrooms she'd had in that "nurturing" elementary school—filled with guinea pigs, pictures, music and a buzz of conversation—were the last thing she needed. She also didn't need teachers telling her she could do better, and that all she had to do was try harder—and parents who didn't believe her when she sobbed that she was doing the best she could.

The External Forebrain

As for the series of counsellors and therapists who told us to "back off" and encourage Colette to make her own decisions and live with the consequences, would they have put a disabled person in a wheelchair with no brakes at the top of a hill and said, "Let 'er rip?" Dr. Sterling Clarren, from the University of Washington, who has led the world in creating diagnostic criteria for FAS, originated the idea that "the person with FAS will always need an 'external forebrain.'"

Think of the forebrain as the world's most sophisticated computer, wired by "little grey cells" rather than microchips. The cerebrum, a key part of the forebrain, consists of the frontal lobes, parietal lobes, temporal lobes and occipital lobes, all with different jobs. But when these parts of the brain misfire because of prenatal alcohol, the affected child or adult requires an outside "hard drive" to help with problems in memory, reason and judgment. That external hard drive is generally another person who can assist in a friendly and nurturing way, but it can also consist of many cues: lists, verbal reminders and an environment that provides structure and boundaries.

Will every person with FASD *always* need an external forebrain? "We don't know," Dr. Clarren told me. "Most adolescents with FAS move through their resentment of outside assistance, and by their twenties, many are grateful for this help. By adulthood, the external forebrain is frequently not a parent, but a partner, friend or advocate."

When I was in the depths of despair about Colette, my grief therapist Dr. Lynne Thurling told me about the "maturational brain spurt" that takes place between eighteen and twenty-three, which might help both of my learning-disabled daughters to acquire some missing abilities. Some adults with FASD seem to have managed to build some new circuits in their damaged computers. They may always need an external forebrain for certain activities—handling their finances or accessing resources, for example—but by understanding their disabilities, helped by community support and sometimes medication, they may be able to cope.

SCREAMS

Remove the supports and the child will fail.
—TERESA KELLERMAN, FAS COMMUNITY RESOURCE CENTER,
TUCSON, ARIZONA

Teresa Kellerman, adoptive mother of two mentally disabled young adults, gives full-length workshops on her SCREAMS model of intervention strategies for parents of children and adolescents with FASD and similar disabilities. Simply put, SCREAMS stands for

STRUCTURE: Daily routine, simple, concrete rules.

CUES: Reminders can be verbal or visual, symbols or signs.

ROLE MODELS: Show your children the proper way to act; practise over and over.

ENVIRONMENT: Low sensory stimulation. Small classrooms, organized home, quiet places.

ATTITUDE: *Parents and professionals must understand that the behaviour of the affected individual is not wilful misconduct; it is caused by neurological problems.*

MEDICATION: Helps put the brain chemicals into balance, and can enable children with FASD to better control behaviour.

SUPERVISION: Twenty-four-seven. Every day. Poor judgment and lack of impulse control never go away.

As I began to understand the implications of Dr. Clarren's "external forebrain," Diane Malbin's "paradigm shift," and Teresa's SCREAMS, I couldn't help wondering: what if we had known about these techniques when Colette was four years old and stealing, seven years old and "lazy" in school, fourteen and getting into drugs? Would our outcome have been different? Our experience with her since 1998 has indicated that if we had applied those strategies when she was younger, she and our whole family would have been spared much anguish.

The Fragile Butterfly

Just one of the many letters I received after the *Elm Street* article was
from a parent whose adoptive child had managed to complete school
and survive intact. This letter was from Marion Dawe, mother of
Rebecca Cave, then twenty-six, who had been diagnosed with FAE
three years earlier. Like me, Marion had learned about prenatal alcohol
damage not through the series of professionals she had taken Rebecca
to, but through a television show. Immediately recognizing her daughter's lifetime disability, Marion had found a geneticist who diagnosed
her daughter with FAE. She sent a clipping from the *Kitchener-Waterloo
Record,* showing beautiful Rebecca, with a sparkling smile, interviewed
about the cause of her memory lapses, depression, short attention span
and learning disabilities: "You have no idea of how good it felt to know
it wasn't my fault . . . I always blamed myself. I always thought I was lazy
or unmotivated or just plain stupid."

Adopted at eleven weeks old, Rebecca was a tiny, underweight baby
with severe eating and sleeping difficulties. She didn't start talking until
the age of three and was delayed in almost every other area of her development. "When I look back at her first year, I realize that she was going
through withdrawal symptoms from the alcohol," says her mother.

Rebecca lives in Kitchener, a two-hour drive from Toronto. She and
I began to write to each other and talk on the phone. Eventually, our
families met. Slim, beautiful, articulate and a talented artist, Rebecca is
a nonsmoker and nondrinker and has managed to avoid most of the
secondary disabilities Ann Streissguth and her researchers write about.
Married since 1996, she still battles low self-esteem brought on by years
of difficulty in the school system. Early in our friendship, she wrote a
letter to Colette about her lengthy struggles and her difficulty in keeping friends:

> I stole things, lied and ran away from home. When I reached high
> school, I decided that I wasn't going to put myself out and try to
> make friends, so I kept away and became a loner. My self-esteem suf-

fered. When anything went wrong, I blamed myself. I became the prime target of bullies, which I had dealt with from public school right into high school.

Like Colette, Rebecca loves animals, and she tried a high school co-op placement as a veterinary assistant, but this attempt failed because of her difficulty in following instructions. She decided to join the military but couldn't pass the math test. She lost twelve jobs in the ten years after completing high school, suffered from depression, and when she looks at her journal from those days, "I cry at my despair . . . The words, 'You're lazy,' 'you're unmotivated,' 'you daydream,' or the worst one, 'you're slow,' punctuated my thoughts over and over."

She tried community college, but failed each test, and the other students seemed to pick on her. Eventually, she studied folk art painting, an area in which she excels. She's had some commissions by decorators, one of them a staircase painted with grapevines, hummingbirds and bumblebees. However, the payment received for the time involved means that her folk art will probably never be more than a way to express herself creatively.

But once-shy Rebecca has discovered another talent—public speaking. In 1998 Vicky McKinney of the FAS Family Resource Institute was looking for speakers for a conference she was organizing in Everett, Washington, and I suggested that Rebecca might do well on a panel. Rebecca agreed to go—somewhat anxiously, as other presenters included FAS stars Ann Streissguth and Dr. Sterling Clarren. The "panel" turned into a captivating, sometimes humorous one-hour slide show, in which Rebecca told her story through charming family photographs. Later, Vicky McKinney wrote that she had wowed the Everett audience, and received two standing ovations.

Since that time, she has blossomed into an articulate and confident spokesperson for FASD. After several years of trying, she and her husband, Mike, are now proud parents of two little sons.

Wife, mother and advocate, this former "out-of-tune angel" now has a strong, clear voice. Why did she survive so well, when so many other young people with FASD find themselves trapped in a downward spiral of addiction and crime? Rebecca has intelligent, loving, supportive adoptive parents—but so did every child whose parents wrote to me. Rebecca has been helped enormously by her family's deep faith and her own—but I know many parents who are also devoted members of religious faiths, which their children had rejected by their teens.

A neurologist familiar with FASD might theorize that Rebecca's birth mother was not drinking at the times when insight, conscience, compassion, determination and verbal skills were developing in Rebecca's brain. A person of religion might say that God sent Rebecca to give a message of hope to parents struggling with alcohol-affected children—or to warn the world that no amount of alcohol in pregnancy is safe for the baby. Lacking my own theory, I merely feel grateful to have had the opportunity to watch this tremulous butterfly test her dazzling wings and take to the air.

CHAPTER SEVEN

A Life Full of Misunderstands

I wasn't failing at something I could do. I was just not succeeding at something I couldn't do.
— David Vandenbrink, with FAS, in unpublished
essay, "One Plus One Equals Two"

The textbooks about fetal alcohol rarely mention the wonderful qualities that make many people with FASD endearing—even though we may occasionally feel like throttling them. Because they live in the present, they can be delightful leisure-time companions, and like Colette, many have a wry, offbeat sense of humour. Despite their learning difficulties, people with FASD may be extremely talented in other areas. Colette is one of many whose fearlessness makes them gifted and confident with animals of all sizes. Some are excellent athletes. Others with FASD have artistic ability as poets, painters or musicians, although their attention problems or addictiveness generally get in the way of worldly success. And over and over, I've found them to possess something all too often lacking in so-called "normal" people—an enormous generosity of spirit.

One of these unique individuals is Stephen Neafcy. In 1996, Steve's older sister Nancy saw a television item about fetal alcohol and connected Steve's lifelong learning and behaviour problems with recollections of their mother's drinking in pregnancy. She organized an appointment for Steve, then forty-three, with Dr. Sterling Clarren of the University of Washington's Faculty of Medicine, whose diagnosis confirmed that Steve was struggling with a brain damaged by alcohol before he was born.

Steve's life changed dramatically. Discovering FASlink, he broke out of his shell of loneliness. By early 1997 he was surfing the Net obsessively, finding out all he could about alcohol, addictions, pregnancy and the alcohol industry. Every day he shared his information: useful Internet addresses; articles in online newspapers, magazines and academic journals; and stories from TV public affairs programs. Even more important, Steve's honest and often humorous observations about his own life gave FASlinkers an understanding of FASD that we could never have had without him.

> At age 43, I had been through a life full of misunderstands and I was always confused on everything that I was trying to be taught! I will be the voice of every FAS/E child. (Stephen Neafcy, post to FASlink)

One of Steve's Net discoveries was the bizarre true story of the railroad foreman Phineas Gage, whose personality changed dramatically after a three-foot, seven-inch long iron rod shot through his head in a rock-blasting accident in 1848. Amazingly, Gage survived, but his frontal lobes were badly damaged. He changed from a man who was socially adept, capable and persistent, to a foul-mouthed, irresponsible lout, given to devising grand, impossible schemes. But Gage's personality change indicated to medical science the role of the frontal lobes in determining personality, and neurological researchers still discuss this case.[26]

Like Gage's iron rod, prenatal alcohol affects the frontal lobes, but that's only part of the damage it does to the fetal brain. In being able to articulate what it feels like to live with permanent neurological damage, Steve and a handful of other individuals struggling with fetal alcohol spectrum disorders have increased my understanding far better than any textbook. They're the twenty-first century's version of Phineas Gage.

Most adopted children with FASD endure a triple whammy: first the neurological disabilities, then the trauma of adoption, then a community of teachers, social workers, therapists and, worst of all, parents, who fail to understand them. But others affected by prenatal alcohol have endured even more damaging emotional trauma. These are the people Donna Debolt calls "stack attack victims," who grow up in dysfunctional biological families or a series of foster homes, enduring childhoods of neglect, terror, emotional abuse and often physical violence.

During their lives, they will encounter many therapists and social workers who will look at their unfortunate experiences in childhood but fail to consider the permanent damage done before birth. These traumatized children, adolescents and adults are at high risk of winding up in tragic newspaper headlines as either predators or victims.

Some, like Steve, manage to survive—barely but miraculously. Two other adults, survivors of both fetal alcohol effects and extremely dysfunctional childhoods, have also generously contributed to this chapter. They are Fran Valentine of Louisiana, another long-time FASlink correspondent, now in her forties, and Rowena Rowley of Chetwynd, northern British Columbia, Canada, now in her early thirties.

Rowena Rowley

I met tiny, blue-eyed, fair-haired Rowena at a conference in early 2001. Chic in a purple faux-silk sports outfit, she was well-spoken and knowledgable about FASD, and I assumed she was a young professional. Then she told me about her childhood, growing up with alcoholic, physically ill, older parents, and spending her early teens in a series of foster homes. Able to obtain her heartbreaking files through her province's Freedom of Information and Protection of Privacy Act, Rowena generously shared these hundred-odd pages with me.

Born in June 1973, the month when the *Lancet* article first defined fetal alcohol syndrome, Rowena was the youngest child born to Winnie Coakley, then forty, who had previously given birth to five other children by other fathers. Winnie and her husband, Ross, forty-seven, were both alcoholics, and there was a ten-year gap between Winnie's fifth child and Rowena. As Rowena puts it, her older siblings were all "off somewhere." She first encountered the social services system at the age of six months, when a government "home aide" reported that the baby was being neglected because of her physically ill parents' "drinking problem." But over a year later, Rowena was still in the care of her family:

> This child has been under constant medical supervision since birth as she suffers from marasmus [failure to thrive]. She has been under the care of Dr. E., pediatrician. The child seems to be progressing reasonably well, although we still have concerns as to the ongoing care the child is receiving, particularly in light of Mrs. C's problem with the bottle. (Social worker's note, November 30, 1974)

Pages of reports from government social workers describe a helpless, malnourished little girl repeatedly ignored, left alone and neglected while her parents drank themselves into oblivion; the reports also indicate, shockingly, that she was left in her horrible situation for years. On several occasions, police were called by neighbours. When Rowena was three, a nurse attending one of the parents notified children's services of a cut on Rowena's eyelid. Her mother explained to the social worker that Rowena had "thrown a temper tantrum shortly before the nurse's arrival, and part of her routine is to hold her breath." Nobody questioned whether this cut was the result of abuse, although records indicate that Rowena's mother offered several different explanations for the cut eye.

When Rowena was four, a social worker scribbled, "Seems things are deteriorating and probably only a matter of time before child is in our care. Please call RCMP and establish exactly why they decided not to remove child on Dec. 8."

At six, Rowena was taken to hospital by ambulance after "an alleged overdose of Dimetapp." The doctor decided to keep her in hospital, as her mother was drunk, and "the child was below normal development when seen previously at the hospital." Six months after this episode, a social worker writes of a doctor who indicated his belief that her "small stature is possibly caused by mother's drinking in pregnancy—failure to thrive." The worker suggested testing at the Diagnostic Centre, but the doctor felt it was not necessary.

When Rowena was seven, her mother complained to a hospital social worker that "she and her husband are having trouble supervising Rowena. She is all over the neighbourhood." The reports go on and on. Elderly disabled parents who are drinking heavily in the bar when their little daughter comes home from school. Visits from the RCMP. The mother taken to hospital by ambulance, "incoherent and making no sense at all." Rowena was temporarily placed in a foster home, and the social worker noted her excitement at this adventure. Two weeks later, Rowena's mother died, and after a six-month stay in two different foster homes, the tiny eight-year-old was returned to her father.

Although Ross seems to have been perpetually drunk, the situation at home was described as "healthy."

> . . . shortly after noon he would go to the pub have a few beers and arrive home in varying states of intoxication. . . . There were occasions when [he] did come home . . . in such a state that he was sometimes abusive, verbally abusive . . .
>
> I suggested to the Judge that we were working cooperatively with Mental Health branch to provide maximum support services . . . to hold this family together as long as possible. He was very much in agreement. (Social worker's report, April 1981)

The records don't mention Winnie's death or any counselling for Rowena, who was already a year behind in school. For the next four years, her inebriated father provided no care at all. On one occasion, attempting to make macaroni and cheese, he threw a whole block of cheese into a pot to melt.

Rowena was now approaching her tenth birthday, and like many females with FASD she matured early. She had problems in school; her teacher was concerned "about her bursting into tears at various times," and she found it difficult to complete assignments. The child care worker reported that she had "poor hygiene habits, little or no awareness of her 'femaleness,' no friends, and few recreational habits." It's not hard to understand those frequent tears at school. The undiagnosed prenatal alcohol damage made it hard for her to process information, and new female hormones were surging through her system; she was malnourished, lonely, "not properly dressed for school" and was "laughed at by the other children." Her father continued to deteriorate, mentally and physically; in that twelve-month period, Rowena experienced three child care workers.

In 1984 her current child care worker complained that eleven-year-old Rowena was living mainly on cereal, and her father was usually drunk or absent. The situation was spooky: Ross had kept nearly all of his late wife's possessions and maintained the house just the way it had been at her death, four years earlier. The frustrated child care worker—the third one that year, and seemingly the only worker in the files who truly connected with the little girl—hand-wrote a note, and underlined it: "<u>I have real concerns about Rowena's father's alcohol problem.</u> . . . Rowena talks about being lonely. . . . There's not much company at home and she alienates kids her own age. She's bossy and whines a lot." The worker wrote that Rowena enjoyed group activities, particularly gym night, and was a willing worker. "She mostly likes to talk, which we do a lot. She feels good when we talk about cleanliness and the next day she shows me clean, shiny hair. She worries about her clothes being inappropriate and has welcomed my invitation to learn to sew some clothes of her own . . . She likes hugs a lot and gives many back."

In August 1984 Ross fell downstairs and hit his head. He wound up in a seniors' home with bouts of memory loss in which he didn't recognize Rowena. (He died in 1991.) Rowena was made a government ward and placed with the Browns, fundamentalist Christians with two biological children and three other foster children. The Browns sent her to the religious school that the other children attended. Aged twelve and a half, in sixth grade, she was performing at grade three level, and described as "somewhat of a handful, behaviour-wise."

> I'd look at the store manager and steal right in front of him. I was massively crying out for help—I wanted attention. I wanted someone to love me and say, 'I love you.' Nobody was willing to give it to me. I allowed the police to come and take me away.
>
> One day [my foster mom] said, "What do you want me to do to you?" I said, "Ground me, discipline me, be mad at me, do something but don't just stand there." She said, "You're too old for that now."

Rowena remained with the Browns until she was eighteen, when her lying, stealing and skipping school became impossible for her foster family. One day one of her foster siblings told her, "Well, nobody likes you in this house. Mum doesn't even love you."

Still in pain at the memory, Rowena remembers asking her foster mother if she liked her, "and she said, 'No, I don't, I don't even love you.' I said, 'Fine, fuck you, fuck you all, I don't need you.' I wanted to kill myself, and that's when I started my *suicidal raid* [suicide threats]."

Rowena tried showing signs that she needed love and attention, but her burned-out foster family had stopped caring. Eventually, she told her eleven-year-old best friend, "this will be the last time you will see me." The friend called her parents, who were there in a flash. The suicide threat led to a psychiatric assessment, and a diagnosis of fetal alcohol effects by a psychologist, Dr. Julianne Conry.

Now in her early thirties, Rowena is fighting hard to have a normal life. Living on disability support, she has always avoided drugs and alcohol. Attempting to build a normal family for herself, she married young. Her husband's background indicates probable fetal alcohol damage. It was a destructive union. They had two children who were removed by child protection authorities in 1998—a daughter and son, then aged three and two. Neglected and abandoned as a child, Rowena had left her young children at home alone on several occasions, and neighbours had informed the authorities.

She has made huge efforts to learn about proper mothering, and to build a "circle of support" in her community, in order to be allowed to raise her children. The key member of this circle is her partner of several years, Richard Harris. In February, 2003, a family court judge finally granted the couple permanent custody of her now school-age children.

Steve Neafcy

Twenty years older than Rowena, but like her the youngest child in a large family, Steve, the fourth child of James and Stella Neafcy, was born in 1953 in a working-class Roman Catholic neighbourhood in Philadelphia. His father, James Neafcy, a pipefitter, had emigrated from Ireland as a young boy. Steve's older brother, Jim, born in 1942, died in 2002. He also has two older sisters, Nancy (born in 1938) and Mary (1951).

Steve's father was a heavy drinker, prone to rages and abusing his children, but Steve has only fond memories of his mother, whose drinking never became apparent until later in life. Forced to drop out of school in eighth grade, James was fanatical about correct speech and grammar, and passed the Irish way with words on to his children. Steve has an intelligent and charming "gift of the gab," but like most people with fetal alcohol disorders, his verbal skills have never been reflected in academic achievement.

> In first grade, he got a broken ankle after jumping off a wall, and had to repeat a grade. Second grade, he repeated. Third grade, he did poorly. Fourth grade he describes as having done very nicely, but really about the same as last year. In my interview with him, he stood and shifted feet constantly. (Psychiatric assessment, 1965)

"My school years were hopeless," Steve adds. "I could not retain anything, my handwriting was unreadable, and the teachers would have a girl sit beside me and help me write my notes. I always puppy-loved every one of those girls."

His sister Mary recalls an event at Holy Innocents Grade School when she was hauled out of her sixth-grade classroom by the nun who taught Steve, then eight and repeating grade two. Unaware of Steve's allergies, the nun made Steve get down on his knees and beg forgiveness for his constant sniffing in class, then angrily demanded that Mary inform her parents of Steve's disruptive behaviour.

> When a group of us got together I felt strange like I was from another planet and I didn't know how to act. So instead of making a fool out of myself I remained quiet and went with the flow . . . Whether it was right or wrong, I went along with it as everybody else was doing it. (Steve Neafcy, post to FASlink)

> His favourite TV program, he stated, is "My Favorite Martian" and describes it as "a man comes down from another planet. He is able to make things go up and down, and somebody carries him around all over." (Psychiatric assessment, 1965)

Eleven-year-old Steve felt as alien as the Martian. Unfortunately, the only magic he could perform was making money disappear from his mother's purse, which often resulted in corporal punishment from his father. Outside the home, the little boy had a few friends, "but it seemed I never fit in."

Like Rowena, Steve lied and stole. Shoplifting gave him a sense of achievement, and a high that lasted until he was outside the store. "I would enter a store without any intention of stealing, but an urge would come over me to take something, whether I needed it or not."

> This is an eleven-year-old boy in 4th grade who enters with a chief complaint of nail-biting, nightly bed-wetting, poor marks in school,

who has developed some nervous habits such as soiling and tics. Mother is described as a worrywart, father described as a dictator who insists upon proper dictionary English and states that the strap is a cure-all for everything . . .

Father . . . is drunk several times a week. He is self-punitive and thinks that all of the problems of his family are his fault . . . Mother gets very angry at Stephen, frequently wants to shake or strap him, but doesn't. Instead, she begs him and this usually fails.

Mother is afraid he is retarded. There is some question of concrete thinking in this boy. There is one instance of looking at a knife and backing away from it and saying that it hurts his eyes. When he was about 5 or 6, this took place . . . If true, this is a frightening example of concretion that might well be a harbinger of future psychosis. (Psychiatric assessment, 1965)

There may have been another reason for Steve's terror: it is possible that he was threatened with a knife by one of the neighbourhood bullies, or even his father in one of those frequent alcoholic tantrums. Steve's sister Mary has vivid memories "of the two of us holding each other and crying when Daddy was on a rampage." Mary also remembers their father "baiting you to do something he knew you would screw up, then . . . beating you in a terrifying rage."

Growing up was like hell—I always knew I was different but never knew why. I was a very slow learner, never fit in with my peers, made up stories just to try and fit in and lied all the time for no reason.

When Steve was thirteen, he began going to Alateen, where he "learned a lot about alcoholism and started to understand my father and his problem." At fifteen he dropped out of school and found a job at Sears Roebuck, filling telephone orders in the customer catalogue department. Things went well for three months, until one terrible morning in 1969 when Steve, feeling like "a big shot," put on a tie and headed down the stairs. His father stopped him and criticized his tie; Steve angrily tore off the tie and stormed off to work.

At work, he calmed down and phoned home to apologize to his father. His mother answered, and Steve asked her to tell his father he loved him. That night he learned that his mother had looked for his father and found him dead in the basement. He had shot himself in the mouth with a rifle. In a suicide note, he blamed himself for his family's problems and told them his death was "a gift" to them. "The loss of my father at that time of my life was almost too much for me to endure," Steve says.

> I have nothing to stop me from having inappropriate behaviour— that was taken away from me before I was born! I was always asking little girls to come into my garage and asking them to pull their pants down. As I grew older my mind kept the same disire of the little girls! I could never figure why I keep my disire for little girls, I had Girlfriends my age but thought of little girls a lot.

This post to FASlink horrified many readers. Ann Streissguth's study on secondary disabilities indicates that during their lifetimes, about 50 percent of males with FASD will commit sexual offences, most often sexual touching and sexual advances. "Being a victim of violence increases the odds of sexually inappropriate behaviour fourfold," her study says.

Unfortunately, because people with FASD are emotionally far younger than their chronological age, they are often attracted to children. Now in his early fifties, Steve profoundly regrets the two incidents in adolescence in which he sexually touched a neighbourhood girl many years younger than himself. The young woman spent many years in psychotherapy as a result, and he realizes there is no way of making amends to her and her family for the anguish he caused.

From his late teens to his early forties Steve's life was an endless series of disasters. After attempts at vocational rehabilitation and the General Equivalency Diploma program, he joined the United States Army in 1971, and received an honourable discharge within three months, on the grounds of "not meeting physical standards at the time of enlistment." A series of dead-end, low-paying jobs followed—dishwasher, busboy, janitor, porter—and at twenty he married plump, pretty, brown-eyed Sally. By 1974, they had two young daughters, whom Steve adored. Sally was the family breadwinner. Steve's verbal skills and charm meant he could always get a job, but keeping it was a problem. Then one day he put a quarter into a slot machine in a drug store and won $1373. After that, "I got the fever and got it bad—started losing a lot and stealing and lying and doing anything to get money to gamble."

Sally tried everything to help her young husband: psychiatrists, religion and eventually divorce. The final decree was granted on April 1, 1980, and he lost all rights to see his daughters, now adults in their thirties. He has had almost no contact with them since that time.

The next fifteen years of Steve's life read like something out of the *National Enquirer*—he bounced back and forth from jail to various mental institutions, and was diagnosed with an assortment of mental illnesses. He'd lost his wife and children, and was unemployable, living on Social Security Disability. His beloved mother had remarried—to a man who hated Steve with a passion. The church where he had found comfort was also pushing him aside, and he was briefly sucked into a strange cult called the "Rising Sun Fellowship."

He spent most of the time between 1980 and 1984 in jail for a series of petty thefts, mostly shoplifting food and clothing. Seemingly without conscience he also stole, even forging cheques from a friend who had invited him to share his apartment. "Jail for me was nothing but a speed-bump until my uncontrollable urges took over."

Steve often spent six months or more in jail, waiting to go to court, as his fed-up family members refused to post bail. "I would be shackled waist, hands and legs to about five to seven other inmates. We would get transported to court in a van, and often spent all day waiting for nothing—then be sent back to jail and do the same thing all over the following day."

> When I was put into the same cage as rapists and murderers and just plain bullies I was in danger, scared to death. . . . Other inmates would

steal your meals and the jailers would do nothing about it. You had to use the bathroom in front of everyone, and there were twelve of us in one large cell. You had to watch out in the shower 'cause another cell-mate would try and have sex with you. . . .

In 1985 Steve joined Gamblers Anonymous and reunited with his mother. Despite having been jailed close to a dozen times for theft, Steve still felt compelled to steal—even from his mother. Disasters continued. A second "divorce" (he discovered at the time of divorce that the Nevada "judge" had never filed the marriage license), being hit by a car while crossing the street in 1990, and having his leg permanently damaged as a result. Worst of all, in 1995, the death of his mother—his greatest source of unconditional love.

But his sister Nancy, now in Washington State, had been reading about fetal alcohol syndrome. She suggested that he move to Washington and seek a diagnosis from Dr. Sterling Clarren. By using his small inheritance, and helped by family members, Steve was able to live in a mobile home near his sister's home. Nancy managed to obtain past medical records and supply some childhood photos, which are essential to diagnosis. In her teens when Steve was born, Nancy informed Dr. Clarren that their mother drank regularly each night during pregnancy, as many as four drinks per occasion.

There were no records of Steve's size in childhood, and as an adult, his height and weight were within normal limits. But in examining Steve's face and baby photos, Dr. Clarren saw several indicators "compatible with alcohol exposure"—short palpebral fissures (eye sockets), and in childhood, a flattened philtrum and thin upper lip. A previous CT and EEG had shown brain abnormalities that could indicate alcohol damage. His IQ was in the low normal range.

Dr. Clarren diagnosed "Static Encephalopathy—Alcohol Exposed" sometimes also known as FAE, ARND, or partial FAS (pFAS):

Stephen has many behavioural problems which are typical of individuals with organic brain damage. He has problems with planning and needs help organizing daily tasks, does not understand the concept of time, and cannot manage money. He has generally difficulty carrying out multi-step tasks . . . problems with behavioural regulation and sensory motor integration . . . poor management of anger, mood swings, impulsiveness . . .

He has demonstrated many antisocial types of activity including lying, stealing, and inappropriate sexual behaviour. In spite of his normal IQ score, he has shown problems with poor memory, slow ability to learn new skills, inability to learn from past experiences, and has had problems recognizing the consequences of his actions. . . .

Dr. Clarren looked over past psychiatric evaluations assessing Steve as having personality disorder, dissociative disorder, depression and schizophrenia, and concluded that "there seemed to be an organic component to his behaviour and he doesn't fit easily into the usual psychiatric categories. . . . Stephen's learning problems and difficulties were never well understood, and . . . this obviously can engender a good deal of depression, anxiety, and even psychotic-like behaviour." Dr. Clarren felt that what Stephen needed most was "for his family to understand the nature of his chronic and continuing disability" and that he be able to live in a "structured and supportive assisted living environment." But the conditions he recommended are virtually unavailable anywhere in the world for adults of apparently normal intelligence struggling with FASD.

Steve's family is typical of countless others. A man who loves his wife and children, but is in the grip of alcoholism, given to violent rages when drinking. A wife or partner in terror who winds up drinking with him, and unwittingly damages a child or children. Steve's three siblings were seemingly not damaged by their mother's drinking: all were university graduates with successful professional careers. Possibly Stella drank less or not at all with her older children, or possibly her liver was healthier and able to better process the alcohol when she was younger.

All his life, Steve had felt like a lonely misfit. But in 2001 a FASlink correspondent began writing to him privately. Barbara, a nurse who was living in Chicago, has an adult child with FASD. She began to appreciate Steve's determination, insight, wry humour and affectionate nature, and welcomed his emotional support by e-mail and phone at a difficult time in her own life. Several cross-country visits ensued, and after a year-long courtship they were married on December 7, 2002.

"I see him as a light-bearing miracle," Barbara wrote to me after they had become engaged, touched by "his warmth, tenderness, whimsy and wisdom." I looked on at a conference on FAS in Saskatoon in May 2003, as the couple made their speaking debut, charming the audience with their knowledge, humour and loving affection. Those of us who care about these two special people—and would never have matched them up—hope they can make this unusual relationship last.

Fran Valentine

All I ever knew my whole life was, I needed a coat, well, I knew how to steal a coat. When you have to survive and you've got your mother drunk and passed out on the bed, you're 8 years old, you don't know what the hell's going on, there's no dad there and you're in a basement apartment on East New York Avenue . . .

A photograph on the website www.fasstar.com shows tall, slim, attractive, auburn-haired Frances Valentine of Mandeville, Louisiana, with her two young adult daughters, looking far younger than her actual age (late forties). Funny and articulate, Fran also sounds half her age, with a Midwestern American accent, tinged only slightly by her Brooklyn roots and a quarter-century as a southerner. As with Steve and Rowena, her verbal skills and sense of humour mask the profound learning disabilities resulting from fetal alcohol.

Born in Brooklyn in 1955, Fran was the only child of her parents' marriage. Her classically beautiful but mentally ill mother came from a large, proud, ambitious family of Italian immigrants; her father was a blond, blue-eyed "Scottish gentleman."

My mother was born schizophrenic into a family that would stick her in the corner with a glass of wine and tell her to quiet down. She was a problem, she was a trouble-maker, they had ten kids, they were immigrants from Sicily settling in America. How can you hold anything against people who didn't know?

Fran's earliest memory is of "sitting on a toilet, watching my parents rolling by fighting with each other, like a tumbleweed—throwing stuff, breaking stuff." Fran can't remember a single peaceful moment with her parents. "It was just so chaotic. Even when they were going to family gatherings, my mother and family were outcasts—my cousins all used to tease me like crazy."

> [My mother] was always very destructive, nasty, mean. It wasn't just the alcohol; that's the way she was born, when you're schizophrenic, that's the way it is. She was always doing weird stuff, she could be so nice and then Bam! Bam! Bam! She'd be banging me around . . .

Her father was a salesman, and her mother worked part-time at Macy's, when not using wine as medication, or "in and out of jails and hospitals." When Fran was eight, her parents separated, and her father's many women friends became far more important than his young daughter. One New Year's Eve, her father dropped Fran at her mother's apartment, to go off with a woman he'd picked up hours earlier at the American Legion. As Fran's mother was drunk and passed out, he broke a window to let Fran in. Coming to, Fran's mother furiously dragged Fran to a corner café, began to be physically abusive, threw dishes and hit Fran so hard that stitches were required. A waitress called the police, and at the police station, Fran was befriended by a woman officer, while her mother, in a white straitjacket, was "tied to a chair and banging up and down and yelling for her mother." Fran still has the photo of herself wearing the woman officer's badge.

Fortunately, her namesake, "Aunt Fran" (her mother's sister), loved the little girl. She lived for a year and a half with Aunt Fran on Long

Island, but her estranged parents snatched her back, accusing her aunt and uncle of kidnapping her.

> There were times when my father would be having sex in the other room with some woman, and I would hear everything he was doing. Or he'd leave me alone for two weeks at a time. He'd wonder why I didn't do good in school, but I never had anybody there to take care of me.

Fran recalls that she "was poor in schoolwork, poor in reading, always ended up being "recommended" (a conditional, generally undeserved "pass" used in the fifties and sixties). Fran lived in a series of informal foster homes, and in one of these she was sexually abused by a boy who lived there. Like Rowena and Steve, she felt compelled to lie and steal:

> I'd just see a boxful of jewellery and I wanted it. I learned what I had to do to get what I needed. I spent many lonely nights in front of a TV set. I was always having problems with relationships and friends. I always told everybody that my mother was dead. I even made up a brother who died in Viet Nam.

When she was fourteen, her Aunt Fran rescued her again, and this time she lived with her loving aunt for three years. Fran believes her two brief periods of normal living with her aunt may have saved her life. "She tried her best with me. She couldn't even get me to wash my hair. I hated baths—would draw the water but wouldn't get in the tub . . . I wouldn't wear underwear—to this day I have to force myself."

At seventeen Fran dropped out of high school, and went to work at an insurance company. A year later, escaping from a destructive relationship, she fled to Florida to study hairdressing—breaking the cycle of addiction and abuse that had destroyed her nuclear family.

> Yesterday, I was depressed (wasn't because of my family) I felt outta it, low. My brain thoughts are slow and spelling words is even harder. My thyroid isn't working take medicine for this . . . I cut my self and

130

never know it, I get black and blues easy . . . I never feel my periods or do I feel normal pain. Its my teeth thats a real problem, at age 14 I had 22 cavitys. Today most of my teeth are fake . . .

Every day of her life, Fran battles numerous physical and mental health problems, but of the three people interviewed in this chapter, she has managed to lead the most stable adult life. In Florida at eighteen, she met and married John, a young mechanical engineer. She and tall, red-headed John have been together more than twenty-five years, and have raised two tall, bright, red-headed daughters. Fran loved being a mother to her little daughters, and as young adults they still laugh about the time Mom convinced them there were gnomes in their yard, constructed a treasure map and buried trinkets in a nearby park. "I was always imagining with them, doing crafts, finger painting, papier mâché—I didn't care if they got stuff all over the place . . ."

But her problems often made family life difficult. There was a period when Fran drank heavily, and a wild spending spree when she racked up more than $30,000 in credit card bills. She feels terrible that her daughters "witnessed me smashing things, yelling and screaming, hitting my head." Affected by bipolar disorder, she has twice attempted suicide. "It's more than just a marriage—the man is a hero," Fran says of John, who has instinctively given Fran the "structured and supported" environment that every person with fetal alcohol damage requires.

Shared Experiences

Fran was not alone in finding life too painful to bear: Steve has attempted suicide numerous times, and Rowena has frequently considered it. All three frequently stole as children and adolescents, had severe learning problems, dropped out of school, had difficulties with employment and had parents with diagnosed or undiagnosed mental health problems on top of their alcohol addiction. (It's possible that Fran's mother and both of Rowena's parents were affected by prenatal alcohol themselves.)

In addition to being affected by prenatal alcohol, Rowena, Steve and Fran were all raised in an atmosphere of neglect and violence. As adolescents, both Rowena and Steve lost parents to premature death, and both have been forcibly, painfully, separated from their own children. Both Steve and Fran struggled with enuresis (bed-wetting). Both Rowena and Fran had great difficulties learning about hygiene. Steve and Fran must take numerous daily medications to control their mental and physical problems. None of the three currently uses alcohol or illegal drugs, but Steve's gambling and Fran's spending sprees have caused them and their families great pain. None of the three was diagnosed with fetal alcohol effects until adulthood.

Even today, three decades since the world became aware of fetal alcohol syndrome, a psychiatrist assessing similar families would probably see so many factors contributing to the children's learning and behaviour problems that she would not consider the prenatal alcohol damage, which no amount of therapy can fix. Psychologists and psychiatrists contend with similar multi-problem patients daily, and possibly we should not be surprised that fetal alcohol is rarely considered as a factor in determining mental health problems. But if the permanent neurological effects of fetal alcohol are not recognized, and a "structured and supported living environment" is not provided, no kind of therapy or treatment is likely to succeed.

Steve, Fran and Rowena, who survived fetal alcohol damage and traumatic early years, are unusual in their determination, insight and ethical sense. They don't perceive themselves as success stories, but they are. They are heroes, whose strength and courage demonstrate the brave resilience of the human spirit.

CHAPTER EIGHT

"From a Little Girl I Was Sad Inside"

We have a whole group of women who are drinking alcoholically. We need to find a way to help them understand that they are damaging their children. Then there are the women who are not alcoholic and don't realize that they are still able to damage their child. They drink from a small amount socially to a regular binge amount, maybe once a month. Our society sends so many mixed messages about the use of alcohol that it's really difficult. We close our eyes or wink about our teenagers getting drunk on the weekend, and we don't educate them about the pitfalls. Education has to start with the teenagers— or younger.

—CHRIS MARGETSON, BIRTH MOTHER AND EXECUTIVE
DIRECTOR OF FASAT IN GUELPH, ONTARIO.

In early 2000 I assisted a journalist who wrote a wonderful investigative article about FASD for a newsmagazine. Her research was thorough, and she checked every fact with me before submitting her copy to the editor. When the issue was published, the cover showed a beautiful little girl with FASD.

The cover line, however, dismayed both of us. It read: "The Sins of the Mothers." Did the drinking mothers get pregnant by immaculate conception? Did they drink alone through nine months of pregnancy? Who sold them or their partners the alcohol? Who benefited from the sale of this alcohol?

To those of us who are not addicted to alcohol, the solution to the problem seems easy. Why don't pregnant women just stop drinking, and why don't women who drink use adequate birth control? *Why won't these women behave responsibly?* Unfortunately, many of us still view alcohol addiction as an individual moral issue, rather than a serious health concern in a society that encourages alcohol consumption.

Research by Dr. Sterling Clarren and his associates at University of Washington indicates that the problem can't be eliminated by telling women not to drink in pregnancy. In a five-year study, the Seattle researchers developed a profile of eighty birth mothers of children who had been identified with fetal alcohol disorders in one of the Washington diagnostic clinics. Eighty percent of these children were living with adoptive or foster parents, so the researchers required the assistance of social service agencies in seeking out the mothers, guaranteeing confidentiality to participants. The birth mothers were "predominantly Caucasian, closely resembling the racial distribution of Washington State, with a slight over-sampling of Native Americans." The researchers discovered that

- most had begun drinking by age fifteen or earlier;
- 79 percent came from birth families in which at least one parent had an alcohol problem;
- 95 percent had been physically or sexually abused during their lifetimes;
- 96 percent had been diagnosed with mental health disorders—the most common being post-traumatic stress disorder (77 percent);
- 73 percent of the live births reported were unplanned;
- 61 percent had not completed high school;
- 59 percent had a gross annual income of less than U.S. $10,000 when interviewed; and
- 46 percent were living on some form of government assistance.

The four most common reasons for not seeking alcohol treatment were:

- not wanting to give up alcohol (87 percent);
- fear of losing their children (42 percent);
- lack of child care (40 percent);
- a partner who did not want them to go to treatment (39 percent).

Of the eighty women interviewed, forty-one reported that they were abstinent by the time their child was diagnosed with prenatal alcohol damage.[27] Most of the women you will meet in this chapter are now abstainers. Two could never have been described as alcoholics or even heavy drinkers, but they, too, unwittingly damaged their children by drinking in pregnancy. Both seldom drank, but consumed many drinks on a few occasions before they realized they were pregnant. Just one episode of four to five drinks over the course of a few hours is defined as a "binge" and can wreak havoc on the developing brain of the fetus.[28]

Mercedes Alejandro of Houston (introduced in chapter 5) is a health research coordinator. She rarely drinks, but now knows that her two episodes of social drinking in early pregnancy were binges, according to professionals working with FASD. Her former husband was a heavy drinker, and before she realized she was pregnant, "we went out to celebrate his new job." Petite, weighing 115 pounds, Mercedes drank three Harvey Wallbangers (each containing two ounces of vodka and one ounce of Galliano liqueur) during the evening. On the second occasion, a tense dinner at the home of friends, Mercedes drank so much she vomited and had to lie down. She did not drink again in pregnancy.

Now a young adult, her son Nicholas, diagnosed with fetal alcohol effects, has an IQ in the low 70s. Mercedes has fought passionately to obtain resources for Nicholas, in both education and planning for his future. He managed to complete high school with the help of a great deal of special education and is fascinated by law enforcement. With Mercedes's help, he has done well at entry-level clerical work for the Houston Police Department.

Mercedes is on the steering committee for the FAS Center of Excellence developed by the U.S. federal government's Substance Abuse and Mental Health Services Administration. Concerned that many U.S. policy planners view FASD as a Native American problem only, she works hard at informing women of Hispanic, Afro-American and Caribbean origin, and other urban women at risk, about the dangers of drinking in pregnancy.

Bright, articulate and well-educated, Mercedes nevertheless partly fits the Clarren team's profile of birth mothers of alcohol-affected children. Her father was an alcoholic and physically abused her mother, and both of Mercedes' former husbands are alcoholics. "I think the typical battering person is controlling, and so when I got into a relationship it felt comfortable, because that's all I had ever known."

"Liz," an elegant marketing executive and mother of a young adult daughter, Susie, does not fit the University of Washington profile at all. Early in her marriage she attended four summer celebrations in four weeks: a graduation party, a wedding, a fortieth birthday and a July 4 party. She rarely drinks, but on each of these occasions she had four or five drinks over the course of several hours, while consuming food. After learning she was six weeks pregnant, she stopped drinking altogether. Baby Susie was born normal and healthy, with an APGAR of 10, but as she grew older, her learning and behaviour problems became a constant source of family turmoil.

After seeing a TV show about fetal alcohol effects when Susie was fifteen and veering out of control, Liz sought a diagnosis for her tall, red-headed daughter. On the basis of baby photos showing early facial features, certain mild health problems, neuropsychological tests and Liz's recollections of those four elegant parties, the diagnosis was "static encephalopathy—alcohol exposed" (a.k.a. FAE/ARND/pFAS). Like Mercedes, Liz now spends many volunteer hours getting across the message that research cannot establish a safe level of alcohol in pregnancy.

There may be many other "moderately drinking" affluent women whose unwitting exposure of their children to alcohol effects has resulted in academic problems and acting-out behaviour. These children may have been diagnosed as having attention deficit hyperactivity disorder (ADHD) or learning disabilities. Such families can often afford the small, structured classrooms of a private school, enabling their children to graduate. Many of these women and their partners will go through life wondering about the errant gene that made one child "different" from his successful siblings or cousins. Still other women may secretly wonder if their children's problems were caused by the "moderate" amounts of alcohol they consumed in pregnancy. They may ponder this possibility in the middle of the night, after their intoxicated teenager has once again smashed up the family car. Then they put the thought away, forever unspoken.

Unlike Mercedes and Liz, who were strictly social drinkers, the four women whose stories we will look at next are in recovery from alcoholism and substance abuse. They grew up in financial situations ranging from extreme poverty to affluence. But the life profile of each one resembles that outlined by the University of Washington researchers. They have courageously told their stories for this book, using their real names, hoping to save other mothers and children from the preventable tragedy of FASD.

Kathleen Mitchell

When I tell my story, I know that these things happened, I know that they're true and accurate, but it's really hard for me to believe, because they are absolutely 100 percent opposite of who I am by nature. It's a really hard thing to envision that I could have ever done these things, and the really strange part of addictive disease, and one of the things we try to educate women to do, is to separate themselves from their disease.

Kathleen (Kathy) Tavenner Mitchell, now spokesperson for the Washington-based National Organization on Fetal Alcohol Syndrome (NOFAS) traces her alcoholism through her father's family. Her paternal grandfather, a federal congressman from Ohio, died of liver disease in his fifties, although "we had no idea that was alcoholism. And my mother also had alcoholism in her family, but it was always looked at as being *Irish.*"

Fifth of seven children, pretty blond Kathleen frequently found herself emotionally neglected by both parents, mostly because of her father's drinking, rages and all-night partying, but also because her mother "was totally overwhelmed, beaten down. Anyone who lives with an alcoholic winds up physically ill, with depression, and isolated, and that was my mom." Kathleen points out that her father's behaviour was the result of the disease of alcoholism. He stopped drinking in 1981, and died in 2001, after twenty years of sobriety during which his wife, children, grandchildren and great-grandchildren enjoyed loving relationships with this gentle and nurturing man.

But during Kathleen's traumatic childhood, "there would be fighting and arguing and bottles being broken. The next day there would be no mention of it." Like many children with alcoholic parents, Kathleen experienced "role reversal": she had to act as the parent of her father and mother. "I worried all day about my mom and little sisters—rushed home from school anxious and sweaty to make sure they were safe."

> I started smoking cigarettes as a kid and drinking, and I had all the early signs of addictive disease when I first used—a high tolerance, blackouts—so I was always a "good drinker." So it was a good thing to be an alcoholic when you were a kid. In the early stages, it's almost an asset 'cause you can drink more than other people, with less of an effect—you're a good party-er.

As a teenager in the late 1960s and early '70s, Kathleen tried alcohol and street drugs—marijuana, LSD, mescaline and amphetamines. Her rock star heroes, Jimi Hendrix and Janis Joplin, were shooting heroin, so why not? She also began experimenting with sex, and in 1971 found herself pregnant, at sixteen. Because of family pressure, she and her boyfriend quickly got married.

Kathleen stopped drinking and using drugs while she was pregnant, but their apartment in a Washington suburb was "a little hippie pad" with black lights and a Turkish hookah pipe, where her high school friends could smoke marijuana. Her husband had a job, and Kathleen went to school half time and worked part-time as a bookkeeper for her parents' restaurant. After giving birth to normal, healthy Danny, "I dressed him up in little blue jeans and tie-dyed shirts, and when he was nine months old, I got pregnant again."

Then her life fell apart. Her husband was arrested, and Kathleen dropped out of school. Living on welfare, stressed because of her husband's approaching court date, Kathleen drank wine throughout her pregnancy, to relax.

> This was a time when they used to give alcohol IVs to women to prevent miscarriages. I'd heard that if you drink a beer a day, it makes your baby big and fat. I thought of it as a nurturing thing, drink a beer, drink a glass of wine, it's really good for the baby's blood— whatever the hell that meant.

Her baby, Karli, was born in 1973 and seemed healthy and normal. When she was six weeks old, Kathleen's husband was sentenced to a long-term therapeutic community for his drug problems. Kathleen moved into her mother's basement and became "a teenager out of control. I was eighteen years old, and I had two children."

Her husband was released two years later, and for the next three years she tried to save their marriage, "never understanding that addiction was a disease and alcohol was part of it . . . if I wasn't using heroin, I thought I was doing great." Kathleen's energy was spent on trying to survive, finding apartments, paying bills and attempting to keep her husband out of jail. A third child, Erin, was born in 1977, and as she had done with her son, Danny, Kathleen stayed clean in pregnancy. In 1978 she left her husband.

"For all of those years, I had focused on his addiction, never understanding that I had my own addiction going on. I think that's typical of women who drink—they usually have a mate who drinks worse than they do. I was the person who made sure the kids got to the doctor and had their lunch money . . . made sure we had the welfare or the food stamps." But like Kathleen as a child, her little son, Danny, became the parent. He "would sit there while I smoked cigarettes and would start to fall asleep, and be nodding out in a high, and he would make sure I didn't set the couch on fire."

A school dropout, mother of three, distraught over her broken marriage and with her self-esteem "ripped apart," Kathleen quickly married a man even more addicted than her ex-husband. Spiralling downward, she neglected her children even more, leaving them with her mother for months at a time. Addicted to heroin, she ended up on methadone maintenance. She became pregnant twice, and both babies—first a son, then a daughter—died shortly after birth. Kathleen is certain that "both of those babies died as a direct consequence of my untreated addictive disease . . . but it wasn't pointed out to me, and treatment was never suggested."

Shortly after her infant daughter's death, her marriage broke up, and Kathleen sank into despair. But her father had earlier completed treatment for his alcoholism and now understood that his daughter, too, was living with the disease of addiction. Both parents did everything possible to help, looking after her children while she twice tried detox and treatment—and twice relapsed. It took a tough counsellor named Big Norman, a recovering heroin addict himself, and a blunt, tearful doctor to pull her from certain death.

> I had all these abscesses from shooting Demerol. I had been shooting heroin into my feet, had an extended liver from hepatitis, I was missing teeth—the doctor just sat there and started to cry. She checked my labs, had me hold my liver, and she said, "D'you feel this? You have alcoholic hepatitis. Your liver is swollen. You see these labs? You are dying . . . You have addictive disease and the only thing I can tell you is, you need help."

Driving away, Kathleen's first response was, "What a freak! Why was she crying?" Then the truth hit. "She moved me because I knew she meant it when she said, 'You're dying. If you don't get treatment, you don't have long to live.'"

She relapsed one more time, and then Big Norman managed to get her into a ten-month program in a government-operated, punishment-style "therapeutic community" for jailed addicts. Kathleen had to wear rolls of toilet paper around her neck, "because I was a 'shitty person.'" Makeup and jewellery were forbidden, and inmates had to wear old clothes, scrub floors and do menial labour while being yelled at constantly. But Kathleen knew it was her last chance. Despite the sickness of methadone withdrawal, lack of energy, memory problems and a brain that seemed not to be functioning, she hung in. She has been clean and sober since 1984.

Living with her parents for the next four years, Kathleen attended twelve-step programs, earned her GED, and began taking night classes. "My resumé was shooting dope, drinking, blackouts, homelessness—I began working in the field of addictions because no one else would hire me." In 1999 she received a master's degree in human services at Lincoln University in Philadelphia.

When Kathleen had been sober for two years, she went to a conference on infants affected by crack cocaine. "The doctor put up on the screen all the symptoms of what crack babies experience—and I saw Karli." Hyperventilating and feeling sick, Kathleen told herself, "Wait a minute, I didn't use crack. What'd I use? I used alcohol."

Researching fetal alcohol at the library, she learned that Karli's many health and developmental problems as an infant were consistent with FAS. Rigid and difficult, baby Karli had had double hernias, chronic ear infections, difficulty sucking on either the breast or the bottle, excessive hair and a high-pitched scream. She was slow in learning to sit up, crawl and walk, and "never seemed to sleep or eat." As a young child Karli had great difficulty remembering things in school, and the school psychologist said she was "wilfully forgetting them as she was angry at her mother for moving her around all the time."

At nine, Karli had been diagnosed with cerebral palsy and mild mental retardation, but Kathleen now instinctively knew that Karli was living with the results of all of that "healthy" prenatal wine. In 1986 doctors at the child development clinic at Georgetown University Hospital confirmed that Karli, then thirteen, had fetal alcohol syndrome.

Coming to grips with the permanent disability she had unwittingly inflicted on her daughter, Kathleen rapidly found herself on the board of the new U.S. National Organization on Fetal Alcohol Syndrome, NOFAS, and has become a powerful advocate for alcohol-affected children. Enjoying close relationships with her family, she has been married since 1992 to a man she met in the twelve-step recovery program, and child-adult Karli lives with them. "He's the sweetest man that God ever made, and says that if I ever leave him, he gets Karli."

Claudia Park

From a little girl I was sad inside, and felt incompetent. I don't remember ever feeling any love from my mother, all she could say was how horrible I was. . . . I was sexually abused from a very young child, by relatives. I told my mother and she said, "It is normal for men to do that." I suffered more than my share of beatings, of emotional abuse and rapes. . . . I drank to feel adequate, and to give myself courage.

Claudia grew up speaking both French and English in her native province of New Brunswick. Her parents were both heavy drinkers. She believes that some of her own lifelong problems may be the result of undiagnosed fetal alcohol damage, and her long, slim face indicates this could be a possibility. She first wrote to FASlink in the fall of 1997, "My oldest son is afflicted with FAS. I drank alcohol and did drugs during my entire pregnancy. I am an alcoholic, and sobered up when he was about a month old." Her son Francis, then twenty, was on probation for attacking her with a knife. "He has a seizure disorder, both petit mal and grand mal, plus the tantrums. He had great difficulty during his teen years and has turned violent towards me. He blames me for all his problems, and in a sense he is right!"

As a result of her son's assault on her, Claudia suffered an extreme mental breakdown. Helped by a psychiatrist, she recognized that the incident had triggered post traumatic stress disorder, related to a long-forgotten childhood incident in which her mother yanked at her arm so hard that she dislocated it. She now understands why she has spent her entire lifetime feeling insecure. "I grew up never, ever feeling my mother's love."

Sexually harassed by her brother, two years older, she told her mother that he "was doing things to me I didn't like. She said it was normal and to stop being such a 'bad girl.'" When she was fourteen, her grandfather grabbed her sexually, and she became depressed and suicidal. Her mother had her committed to a mental institute.

Claudia never told her father about what her brother had done to her, fearing his reaction. She recalls that her father cried as he signed the papers committing her to Montreal's Douglas Hospital, but doesn't remember much of the three years when she was locked up. Heavily medicated, she was given shock treatment and saw a psychiatrist regularly. When she was allowed out on weekends, she began drinking with friends. "Drinking eased my pain, and it gave me courage."

Her father paid for a course at a private business college; at eighteen, she found a job and signed herself out of the hospital to live with her boyfriend, a musician "who drank and did drugs, just like me." When he physically abused her, she thought this behaviour "was only natural because I thought I had caused the problem." For six years Claudia hung onto her job, blowing her pay on alcohol. Eventually, she dumped the musician, went back to school to complete her GED, and found a new boyfriend, who lined up loaded shotguns and threatened her when she refused to have sex. That relationship lasted two years.

I remember thinking, "Gee, now I have 85 cents, that's almost enough for three drafts!" I never thought about eating or sleeping. I had no

143

home, nor did I care to have one. I hadn't contacted my family in a year, and I didn't even give it another thought. All I wanted was to get high—and stay drunk, period.

By 1975, aged twenty-six, drinking alone, she hit Montreal's version of Skid Row—lower St. Lawrence Street—spending an entire year "drunk or high twenty-four hours a day . . . I lived, worked and craved alcohol day in and day out." In July 1976 her then boyfriend beat, raped and kicked her so badly that she needed medical attention—and in October she learned she was four months pregnant. "Wow, I thought, a baby!"

During her pregnancy, Claudia worked as a waitress in a *brasserie* (tavern), managing to stay sober on the job. Finishing her shift at midnight, she would go to the adjacent night club and order a "healthy" glass of milk loaded with Tia Maria. Binge-drinking in the seventh month of pregnancy, she wound up in hospital with delirium tremens, and two weeks before her baby was due she and his father were married in a "forced wedding." Francis's birth, on March 26, 1977, was a terrifying event. Claudia hemorrhaged; her tiny five-pound baby did not cry, and was wheeled away in an incubator and placed under observation.

She finally saw him twenty-four hours later, and was overcome with love, rocking him for as long as nurses would allow, crying and singing to him, ignoring the social worker who urged her to give up Francis for adoption. She managed to stay sober for twelve days, then binged for the next week. Drunkenly coming out of blackout in a club near her parents' home, she heard someone sobbing, and looked up to see the one person in her family who had never abused her, her father, with tears streaming down his face.

"He kept saying over, and over, 'Give me the baby, give me my grandson!'" Stunned to see tiny newborn Francis sleeping in her arms, wearing only a diaper and T-shirt, Claudia handed him over to her father, who gently wrapped him in a warm blanket and held him close.

Then he told her, "Claudia, I love you with all my being, I didn't know you were so sick. Please for your own sake stop drinking . . . and if you want to continue to be his mother don't ever let me catch you drunk like this again." She hasn't had a drink since.

Francis was diagnosed with fetal alcohol syndrome at birth, but Claudia didn't understand what that meant. He was "undeveloped," with nails missing from his toes and fingers, and his ears were not developed at all. He couldn't suck, trembled most of the time and had numerous seizures, requiring trips to Emergency. By the age of eighteen months, he had been hospitalized four times, and "the Montreal Children's Hospital was our second home."

> I don't know how I could have prevented it, because I didn't know
> how sick I really was, nor did I know that alcohol could cause such
> irreparable damage to my unborn child. I wanted a baby, but not in
> the conditions in which I had him. I wanted a real life . . . with a nice
> home, and love all around me.

Now in his twenties, Francis still struggles with learning difficulties, behaviour problems and rages, all caused by prenatal alcohol. He has problems with employment and frequent encounters with the law. He has occasionally become estranged from his mother. Claudia has attended a twelve-step program since Francis was four weeks old, and now helps other women in recovery whose drinking in pregnancy has damaged their children.

Traci Henke

I thrived on the altered state of mind. I smoked cigarettes from age ten. I liked the burn of alcohol on my throat from the first time I tried it. It made me feel happy . . . it made me feel better.

Traci Henke of Sacramento, California, sent me videos and photos of herself and her school-aged son, Isaac. It seems inconceivable that this gentle, articulate madonna with long brown hair and large brown eyes could have been "living out of a Dumpster" when her child was conceived. But in 1989, in Eureka, California, she and Isaac's father were living on the street, surviving by panhandling and using alcohol and any other drug they could obtain.

Unlike Claudia Park and Kathleen Mitchell, Traci says she was never abused or neglected. She believes her tendency towards addiction was inherited through her father, an alcoholic whom her mother divorced when Traci was nine. Both of her father's parents died of alcoholism, and his mother was mentally ill, as well.

Despite the constant support of her loving mother, a non-drinker, Traci began drinking at ten, and by fourteen she was partying with men in their twenties. Her keen intelligence enabled her to mask her alcohol and drug use both at home and at school. Despite her frequent truancy, Traci managed to graduate from a four-year high school program in only three years.

By 1979, aged twenty-two, she had moved on to hard drugs, and was estranged from her mother. Working full-time for a large supermarket chain, she earned $13 per hour and was "shooting $300 a day in coke, as well as drinking Southern Comfort," and making up the difference by dealing. For the next four years she used cocaine intravenously—miraculously escaping infection—and prevented needle tracks by using Preparation H.

When Traci learned she was four months pregnant, she was terrified. It was 1989, and she was thirty-two. Returning home to Sacramento, she continued to drink as much as a quart of whiskey a day until the last month of her pregnancy, when she quit cold turkey.

Isaac weighed only four pounds, four ounces when he was born, and was diagnosed with failure to thrive. Attempting to stay sober, Traci breast-fed him for the first six weeks of his life, but when her milk dried up she immediately began drinking again. Her mother called child protection services, and Traci drunkenly handed Isaac over to the sheriff. The following day, she woke up stunned and clear-headed: "I finally realized that I was going to have to be clean and sober and live with all those people I hated or I was gonna die."

She was furious with her mother, Isaac's social worker, Nick, and her baby's foster mother, all of whom told her that if they ever saw evidence of drinking, she would never see her baby again. Motivated by the fear of permanently losing her baby, Traci attended a twelve-step program three times a day and volunteered for drug and alcohol testing three times a week.

At the end of three months of sobriety, she was given temporary custody of Isaac. But like almost everyone in early recovery, she had a major "slip"—buying Nyquil for a cold, and drinking several bottles. Discovering that she had a conscience, she called Nick, the social worker, who told her, "I could snag this baby, but I ain't coming. You take care of him." She never drank again.

Rapidly becoming as committed to her twelve-step program as she had been to drinking and drugs, Traci lived on welfare, taking Isaac by stroller to as many meetings as she could fit in, where members took turns holding him. Eventually she was able to return to the work force, and now runs a successful small business.

Traci came dangerously close to slipping again in 1991, when a doctor told her that one-year-old Isaac probably had FAS. She thought about going to the liquor store but instead "went to four meetings back-to-back that night to help me stay sane." Needing an official diagnosis for her own peace of mind and to access services, Traci put Isaac on the waiting list to see Dr. Sterling Clarren in Seattle. Finally, in September 1996, Clarren diagnosed Isaac, who was then six, with atypical FAS, and Dr. Ann Streissguth assessed Isaac's full-scale IQ as 48.

In January 2001 he was assessed again at the Center for Behavioral Teratology, in Scripps Hospital in San Diego. "Unfortunately, even in . . . a loving and stimulating home environment, his general level of functioning is very low," wrote Dr. Brigitte A. Robertson, adding that Isaac would need supportive living throughout his life. "His level of disability is substantial and his capacity to complete even the simplest task without supervision is minimal." Isaac is approaching adolescence as I write this book, but he functions at the level of a preschooler.

Slim and attractive, Traci says she will never get married. "My mom keeps saying, 'I don't want you to end up like me,' but I say, 'What's the matter, you haven't wound up so bad.' I share the life that I have with my son and my mom and my work. I don't know that I want to give up any of these things. The trade-off isn't worth it."

As for guilt: "I hold myself accountable and responsible, and the best way to deal with it is to move on to whatever avenues I can find to help Isaac—and to work. In my sobriety, my work is the one thing I've perfected."

Monica Bourassa

My whole biological family is messed up in some way. My birth dad drinks beer, hair spray, Listerine, and can barely talk because his throat is burned from all this. My birth mother parties every weekend, and has twelve or thirteen kids—from what I see, she doesn't look after them very good.

Still in her early twenties, Monica Bourassa, who has a distinctive round face and dark-rimmed glasses, jumped to her feet and angrily spoke out during a presentation I was giving in Saskatoon. The passion, intelligence and determination that captivated the audience may also have enabled her to survive a hellish childhood and adolescence, similar to that experienced by many North Americans of native background.

Born on a reserve in Saskatchewan, Monica is the youngest woman interviewed for this chapter, and although her birth mother was a heavy drinker, Monica seems to have escaped prenatal alcohol damage. She was adopted at the age of eight months by a mother of aboriginal background and a father of French-Canadian heritage, who already had three biological sons older than Monica. Unfortunately, she was still surrounded by the alcohol and violence that had destroyed her family of origin, and for the next decade she endured "a lot of physical abuse from my mom, and sexual abuse from my adoptive father."

When Monica was ten, she told her adoptive mother about her father's abuse, and wound up in foster care, briefly living in a loving foster home with no alcohol or violence. However, the earlier abuse had permanently affected her, and Monica seemed driven to rebel. When she was thirteen, her exhausted foster parents turned her back to the authorities. The next step was a group home. "I kept running away, and then I got introduced to alcohol. I thought, 'Well, this is fun, it takes me to a place where everything is okay.'"

Monica's first child, a daughter she named Christian-Lee, was conceived in a short-lived relationship that ended soon after Christian-Lee's birth in May 1995. Monica knew about FAS, and did not drink during this pregnancy, but once the baby was born, Monica hit the bars. By now she was seventeen, but looked much older. The baby was removed by social services, and to get her back Monica was ordered to attend an addiction centre. Instead, lonely and scared, she felt driven to return to the bars, quickly discovering that prostitution was an easy way to obtain alcohol. "I sure didn't like myself, my body felt dirty, and I just didn't care any more, because I was alone again, and that was something that I couldn't do—be alone."

Eventually regaining custody of her daughter, she stayed sober until she met Walter, who became the father of her two younger children. "About a month or two into the relationship, he started throwing things at me—a book, a brush . . ." On one occasion, Monica defended herself by stabbing him in the chest with a steak knife. Five months into the relationship, Monica discovered she was pregnant, knew she should quit drinking, but didn't. "By then, I hated Walter, but stayed with him because I was so afraid of being alone."

> When I was pregnant with Tanner, and drinking, I still wasn't willing to admit that I had a problem. I was so ashamed of myself. When I drank, I didn't have those feelings any more. . . . Walter was in and out of jail, and when he was in jail, I drank more, because I couldn't be

alone. I had this great big thing of being alone and not belonging to somebody—not having someone to be my mom and my father, my family—so I'd go sit in the bar.

Monica rationalized her drinking by thinking she would give the baby up for adoption. But as soon as Tanner was born, in July 1998, "I was amazed at how beautiful this child was." Like Claudia Park and Traci Henke, she was instantly smitten with her newborn son, and adoption was out of the question. "I was adopted and I felt lost for a lot of years of my life. I did not want him to grow up angry, feeling alone and worthless."

However, as soon as Monica brought tiny Tanner home, she and Walter began drinking and fighting again, and both children were taken into foster care. Like many addicted women whose children are removed by authorities, she immediately became pregnant with her third child. Because of the high degree of awareness of FASD in Saskatchewan, Monica knew that alcohol in pregnancy is dangerous to the fetus, and secretly feared that her drinking had damaged Tanner. Vowing to stay sober in this third pregnancy, she went to a native treatment program, CHUM (Creative Healing for Urban Members), again deciding to place this child for adoption. And again, the minute she saw Keegan, born in January 2000, she could not give him up.

Determined to break her family's cycle of alcoholism and abuse and overcome her own need for a man, "I decided, I can do this by myself now." She began to understand her own addiction and why she drank—"to cover up a lot of pain from my childhood." She managed to get her children back. Despite shame and embarrassment, she found the courage to tell a counsellor about her heavy drinking when she was pregnant with Tanner. He was diagnosed with full-blown FAS in July 1999, at the age of two.

Monica tells the world that, despite his FAS, Tanner has many wonderful qualities. "He's got a great sense of humour. And he brings life into my home. My other two have their own personalities, but Tanner takes the cake. He's so outgoing and loveable—these kids are lucky to have him as a brother."

Strongly motivated by love for her children, and assisted by a circle of caring aboriginal professional women, Monica is working hard to become independent. Her therapist has been helping her deal with both her painful childhood and knowledge of her large, addictive birth family. She completed her high school diploma in 2001, and hopes to eventually earn a college diploma. "I've learned that I can be alone, and I can make it. That took a long time to learn—being alone was something that I never thought I could do."

> *Mothers who drink are some of the strongest individuals I have ever met in my life. You're looking at survivors. The great percentage of them have been sexually, physically, emotionally abused, lived with abusive mates. . . .*
>
> *These are women who sometimes have been homeless, have not had enough money to pay the rent, or had enough food in the cupboard. These are women who can survive things that most women can never conceive of happening.*
>
> —KATHLEEN MITCHELL

Kathleen Mitchell believes that the almost instantaneous addiction to alcohol that she and the other women describe in this chapter may be the result of genetic programming. If you take a young woman whose biochemistry predisposes her to addiction, and then add the emotional trauma of growing up in a dysfunctional family, should anyone be surprised that this young woman quickly becomes addicted to alcohol or street drugs?

Pregnancy and childbirth made Monica, Traci and Claudia determined to clean up their lives: all were afraid of losing their children to the local child protection agency. In social work lingo, this period is a "teachable moment." The highly successful Birth to 3 Program (now known as P-CAP) developed by Dr. Ann Streissguth in Seattle takes advantage of this window, during which a woman with substance abuse problems may be more receptive to treatment. Similar programs are now being used successfully in many other North American communities. Unfortunately, by the time the mother is helped she has generally given birth to an alcohol-affected child.

Kathleen Mitchell says that birth mothers are no different from other women with addictions, and points out the need for more resources for all women with substance abuse problems, particularly those of childbearing age.

Listening to the tapes of the women interviewed for this chapter, I realized that the problem of maternal drinking in pregnancy cannot be separated from the widespread culture that accepts and encourages frequent and often irresponsible alcohol use. The wine industry has managed to position wine as a health beverage. Beer becomes associated with our favourite sports. Fruit-flavoured coolers attract adolescents sneaking their first drinks. All too frequently, the media portray alcohol consumption as sophisticated and drunkenness as amusing; the tragedy of alcoholism is almost always ignored. TV, our biggest media influence, rarely educates us about the critical public health issue of FASD.

Early in my writing career, I wrote slick and sassy advertising copy for one of the world's major alcoholic beverage companies. Today I wish that every TV advertiser promoting beer, wine or spirits was forced to provide equal time to birth mothers of alcohol-affected children, so that the general public could meet these youngsters, see the pain in the mothers' faces, listen to the regret in their voices. A thirty-second commercial featuring just one of the mothers interviewed here—and her child—would be a strong force in preventing FASD.

CHAPTER NINE

They Come without Cookbooks

It's not something you can do on the side—it's a full-life commitment. They don't accompany us on our life's journey, they sweep us off the path and down their own rocky roads with a flash flood. We grasp at sandbars along the way; find temporary high-ground only to be swept away again by the tidal wave of FASD. Our consolation is that, together, this child might survive those rapids. Alone, they drown along with the sorrows of their birth mothers in the alcohol that has condemned them. Can we teach them to swim? Maybe. Can we keep them alive? Maybe. Can we let go and watch them drown alone? Impossible.

—Claudia Barker, Bastrop, Texas

On the morning of December 31, 1991, Claudia Barker and her husband Kelly were sitting at the breakfast table in their home in Austin, Texas, planning a "boring" New Year's Eve, banging pans with their three school-aged sons. But a few hours later, their evening and their lives would be permanently changed by a tiny baby girl who had been living under a bridge with her teenage mother. A desperate social worker from Child Protection Services called them at noon. Could the Barkers possibly provide emergency foster care *immediately* to a neglected baby?

More than a decade later, Claudia and Kelly Barker are still entranced by their complicated little New Year's gift. Ann Streissguth's secondary disabilities study indicates that, like baby Anne Marie, as many as 80 percent of people with FASD are not raised by their biological parents. Some will be raised by other family members— grandparents, aunts and uncles, siblings or step-parents. Others will be raised by adoptive parents or in a permanent foster setting. All of these children are far more fortunate than the countless alcohol-affected children who will spend their childhood on the move from foster home to foster home.

The Barkers and Anne Marie

Three hours after the emergency phone call, the social workers arrived with three-month-old Anne Marie, whose thick black hair was filled with lice and nits. She weighed only eight pounds, less than Claudia's sons had weighed at birth. "Her little face was squinched up in a frown, and she wouldn't make eye contact." Stiff as a board, the baby didn't move or make a sound. After checking with her pediatrician, Claudia washed the baby's hair with lice-treatment shampoo, and by the time she finished, a great deal had fallen out, leaving bald spots.

The baby ate well, but for two days she didn't make eye contact, move so much as an arm or leg or make a single sound. Her face remained tight-squinched and worried-looking. On the morning of the third day, Claudia walked into Anne Marie's room and said, "Good morning, pretty girl!" The baby made eye contact with her and *smiled.* "I felt a shiver and thought, 'I've got her! There's a person in there!'"

Claudia was hooked.

Social workers had warned that Anne Marie often stopped breathing and turned blue. Fearing sudden infant death syndrome, Claudia felt it was necessary to be with her every moment, and often slept with the baby on her chest to ensure she was still breathing. Because Anne Marie's rigid little body didn't fit into store-bought baby slings, Claudia copied the Korean mothers in the English classes she had been teaching. Making a sling out of soft cloth diapers, she wrapped Anne-Marie on her chest, tight enough so that the baby could feel her heartbeat "and loose enough so that I could see her face when I talked to her." Claudia learned much later that Anne Marie had also suffered from lead poisoning, another cause of neurological damage—possibly a result of her birth mother's sniffing of gasoline booster.

For the next three months, Anne Marie followed Claudia with her eyes, but didn't move or make any sound. "Then she began making a sound of 'eh, eh, eh,' like a kid imitating a machine gun. It was both her cry and her laugh." Unable to tolerate rocking, the baby would withdraw into sleep when overwhelmed with sights or sounds.

Claudia's friends said, "What a good baby!" and "You'd never even know she was here!" But Claudia knew that something was wrong, and when Anne Marie began to throw tantrums around her first birthday, Claudia saw them as a step forward from "her previous method of 'leaving us.'" Heading off "melt-downs" caused by over-stimulus, the Barkers kept Anne Marie out of stores and restaurants because the sights and sounds would overwhelm her.

Attempting to find out the source of Anne Marie's many problems, Claudia took her to a geneticist. He asked the two-year-old to take off her shoes, and when she shook her head, he removed one anyway, and handed it to her. "She whacked him in the crotch with it," says Claudia. "He never liked us after that." At the second appointment, he warned Claudia that "there were no metabolic disorders, no genetic disorders, that this kid was only trouble. And maybe she looked cute now, but she was going to be hell, and I should hand her back to the social worker, and *run* in the other direction!"

Claudia then discovered an excellent program run by Easter Seals, where personnel tested Anne Marie to find out how she could best be taught. Anne Marie, delayed in speech, would scream furiously at Claudia, who would desperately ask, "What do you want me to do?" Easter Seals taught Anne Marie some basic signs, which allowed her to communicate her needs. Many of the rages vanished as Anne Marie quickly began learning the signs and also reading lips: she continues to take in about 80 percent of her speech information from lip-reading. Claudia now recommends sign language for all small children with speech delays, and says that even infants can learn simple signs.

Anne Marie's early experiences as an alcohol-affected child at pre-school were lessons in humiliation. She lasted only two weeks at a half-day program that her big brothers had loved. A little boy kept pulling her long black hair, despite the teacher's repeated admonitions. One day he yanked the tiny girl's hair again, and she furiously knocked him down to the ground, kicked, bit, hit, scratched and yelled, and was pulled off him still kicking and screaming. The boy's mother—another teacher—threatened to resign if Anne Marie didn't leave. Anne Marie is only one of many alcohol-affected children who have been expelled before entering first grade.

Claudia then found an early-childhood program for Anne Marie, through the public school's special education department. The small class of eight was a good fit, but after a year, Anne Marie tested too high to come back. Like many other children and adults with FASD, her disabilities made it difficult for her to participate in the mainstream, but were not considered severe enough to require permanent special assistance.

Before her daughter hit first grade, Claudia put together a detailed package of information about FAS, but "got a teacher whose attitude was, 'I'm going to whip this kid into shape.' It was a horrible first semester."

Anne Marie handles stress by withdrawing, and the teacher's grating voice hurt her ears. The little girl would crawl under furniture to hide or, in cold weather, leave her coat on inside school and pull the hood up over her head. Then the teacher would try to remove the coat. Claudia was constantly receiving notes from the teacher, and Anne Marie would "melt down" every day after school.

She was given a special FM unit to wipe out distracting classroom noise—a device that is often effective with children with FASD. Anne Marie wore headphones, and the teacher wore a microphone, so that the only sound Anne Marie could hear was the teacher's voice. Unfortunately, the teacher didn't bother educating herself about the unit. "She would shout across the room with the microphone on and blast Anne Marie out of her seat—or flush the toilet with the microphone on, sending Anne Marie up the wall."

Everything fell apart the day of a surprise Christmas assembly, which disrupted routine for Anne Marie. After much "rah-rah" yelling in the gym, the class was given a test in spelling, a difficult subject for Anne Marie. When the teacher told them to put their pencils down, Anne Marie didn't hear, and kept writing. The teacher then screamed in her face: "I said, put the pencil down!"

Anne Marie threw the pencil across the room, and the teacher threw her to the floor, with her knee in the screaming six-year-old's back. Finally, she stopped screaming and crawled on her stomach underneath the table. The teacher called the counsellor in, and both women dragged her out by her feet from under the table. Anne Marie went berserk, tipped over desks, threw books and backpacks everywhere. Claudia arrived to find Anne Marie shaking and sobbing, while the counsellor shouted at her to clean up the room. She asked the counsellor to leave the room and quietly began cleaning up the mess, and Anne Marie started to help.

When they had finished, the principal sat Claudia down and brusquely told her: "The slim rewards of teaching a child like this simply aren't worth the challenges she presents. Anne Marie will probably not become a taxpayer." During the next semester, Claudia, experienced in teaching English as a second language, began seeking an alternative for her daughter's education. She looked into private schools, but found they weren't affordable. Neuropsychiatric tests confirmed that Anne Marie had poor short-term memory, and difficulty with math, spelling and abstract or conceptual thinking. In the small community of Bastrop, Texas, where they now lived, there were no other schools or programs. Claudia's only option was to home-school Anne Marie. Like many parents on FASlink, she has home-schooled her daughter ever since.

The Frank Family and Adam

While Anne Marie was quietly becoming a permanent fixture in the Barker household, another adopted child had just arrived in his new home, 3,500 kilometres to the northwest. In rural Alberta, Lynn Frank and her husband, Allan, were enjoying their new son, Adam, a cuddly and affectionate toddler. Lynn and Allan had married in 1979, soon after Lynn had completed her degree in psychology. After learning that Lynn was infertile, they applied to adopt. In the following seven years they adopted Rachel, Jeremy and Marie—born in 1984, 1985 and 1988 respectively—all of aboriginal background.

When Lynn and Allan met sixteen-month-old Adam, they were captivated. As they walked into the foster home, he ran up to Lynn, put his arms up to be held and snuggled up against her. Lynn thought, "This is meant to be, it's love at first sight!" The following day they made the four-hour drive home with him, and he settled in immediately, with no fussing or anxiety. (Lynn now realizes that this quick familiarity can indicate the attachment disorder that so often accompanies FASD.)

Adam's foster mother had warned Lynn that Adam didn't show his temper often, but when he did—look out! However, Allan and Lynn saw no evidence of these rages, and a year later, they finalized the adoption. In the next three years the family would grow beyond their wildest dreams (and against medical science predictions): in 1995 Lynn gave birth to a daughter, Melissa, and in 1997 to twin boys, Joshua and Jordan. Adam and the other children were entranced by these babies.

Athough Adam's temper occasionally surfaced in the form of violent rages, he was generally "a sweet, loving, eager-to-please, affectionate little boy" who charmed friends and neighbours. Proud of her fearless, confident little son, Lynn worried about his occasional tantrums, but failed to recognize them as danger signals.

Adam's kindergarten teachers first described him as a "pleasant, cooperative, polite and helpful little boy"—but then his serious behaviour problems and rages began. "When he went into a rage, a look would come over his face that would make the hair on the back of my neck stand on end. His eyes would narrow and his voice would change to a growl." At six, in one of those rages, he growled at Lynn's brother, "I am going to kill you!" Lynn's brother looked at her, stunned. "I think he means it."

On one occasion at school, Adam threw a tantrum at lunchtime over a tuna sandwich (his favourite). He tore the sandwich apart, threw his entire lunch across the room, and then picked up his desk and threw *it* across the room, while the other children cowered. At this point, Lynn and the school recognized that her son had a serious problem. However, school staff blamed the parents for his behaviour, suggesting various vague remedies, such as: "Spend more time with him," "Boost his self-esteem," "Discipline him more" or "Discipline him less."

Lynn has kept a detailed journal of her son's behaviour and all of the psychologists, psychiatrists, pediatricians and other professionals who became involved with him over the next few years—the psychiatric and pediatric fees paid for by Canadian medicare, the psychologists mainly by Lynn and Allan. Two professionals said that Adam was unable to bond or attach; for the family's safety, they recommended that he be removed from the family home. Lynn and Allan refused to accept this opinion, believing that they had bonded quite well with this cuddly and affectionate little boy. Another doctor told them that Adam was too young to diagnose, but showed signs of paranoid schizophrenia.

Adam, then seven, with an above-average IQ of 106, was diagnosed with FAS in 1996, and the doctor diagnosed both Jeremy (eleven) and Marie (eight) as having FAS as well. Relieved, Lynn thought, 'Well, that explains so much—now all I have to do is educate myself about FASD, and I will be able to help my children.'"

Adam's increasingly frightening behaviour was a huge challenge, even for parents with the Franks' intelligence, education, insight and energy. On one occasion, he took an exacto knife to school and began waving it around and swearing at people. His father locked up all the knives and scissors in the house, but Adam managed to find knives anyway, on one occasion slashing everything in the bedroom he shared with his older brother, Jeremy.

Lynn called one of the province's specialists in FASD—an adoptive mother of two alcohol-affected young adults. Lynn says that the best advice this compassionate social worker could give was to "pack Adam up, take him to the closest social services office, hand him over and tell them it's an adoption breakdown." Stunned, Lynn could not bear the thought of abandoning this little boy, who could also be sweet, charming and wonderful. Nevertheless, the family was under severe stress. Lynn and Allen were also dealing with Jeremy, then thirteen, and Marie, ten, both with FASD—as well as the normal needs of fourteen-year-old Rachel and their three little biological children. "It was like being a triage nurse in a war zone, having to decide who was worth saving and who wasn't," Lynn says. "It is a horrible decision to have to make: *who in your house can you make a difference with?*"

On Good Friday 1998, the Frank family acquired a nine-week-old puppy, a border collie/husky cross. For three days, the puppy never left Adam's side. Watching them frolicking together, Lynn dared to hope this would be a turning point in his life—maybe all he needed was the unconditional love of a dog.

On Easter Monday, Adam asked to go outside and play with the puppy, and Lynn let him go, on the condition that he stayed visible from the window. She watched him play with the puppy for fifteen minutes, turned away for a minute—then looked back outside and was horror-struck. Adam had a large stick and was viciously beating and kicking the puppy. Running outside, she grabbed Adam, asking why he was doing that. "His reply was the classic FAS, 'I don't know.' At that moment I knew in my heart what everyone had been telling me but I didn't want to believe."

Five months later, in September 1998, nine-year-old Adam left their home for good. Untangling themselves from the adoption and their mixed feelings about Adam left the family heartbroken but relieved. Lynn was stunned that Adam quickly lost interest in his adoptive family and immediately began calling his temporary foster mother "Mom." It was just one more manifestation of his underlying attachment disorder.

Transplanted Children

The Barkers are typical of many parents whose "temporary" foster children quickly find a permanent place in their hearts. Some of these foster children will be formally adopted; others for various reasons will not. Many parents can't afford to give up the small subsidy they receive for foster care. For others, adoption is impossible, as many adoption agencies no longer allow parents of Caucasian background to adopt children of other races. Official terms such as "guardian" and "conservator" are sometimes used to describe these people, but their kinship with their transplanted children is engraved in their souls, not spelled out on paper.

There are about 600,000 foster children in the United States, and the North American Council on Adoptable Children website indicates that for 120,000 of these adoption would be a reasonable goal. According to the Adoption Council of Canada, although there are no federal statistics, there are between 60,000 and 80,000 foster children in Canada. Tragically, foster parents generally have no rights where the law is concerned. I've known many foster parents who have lost beloved children they had raised since birth. They watched in despair as wailing, terrified children were given by authorities to dysfunctional biological parents, or to extended family members whose interest seems only financial. During the summer of 2002, a two-year-old boy with full FAS was torn from a loving foster mother who wanted to adopt him, and returned to a twenty-year-old pregnant mother who was also alcohol-affected: within weeks, he had been beaten into a coma by the woman's boyfriend, and is unlikely ever to walk or talk again.

Each of our daughters benefited from being "the baby" in the warm and nurturing Newbigging household until she was made available for adoption. During their long, career as foster parents, Cliff and Dona Newbigging cared for about forty infants, one at a time. They and the many other foster families I have come to know on FASlink have taught me that, for most foster parents, this difficult, often heart-rending work is not something they do for money. Without their devotion and willingness to work for a pittance, child protection agencies around the world would collapse.

Yet even the most loving foster home might not be appropriate for a child with FASD. The alcohol-affected child does best in a calm, structured environment, with much one-on-one attention. Many foster homes are the exact opposite—with several children, they are noisy, cluttered and full of distractions.

Adoptive parents generally have a different set of expectations, as Brian and I did. Adoption agencies may warn that the process of blending a family will not be smooth, but few adoption workers clearly explain to parents the fact that fetal alcohol damage may be present even in children who have not been diagnosed—especially those with family histories of alcoholism. When children have been diagnosed with FASD, the worker may treat the permanent disabilities of alcohol-related brain injuries as a hangover that will go away lots of love. Jo Nanson, a psychologist in Sasakatoon who has specialized in assessment of children with FASD, says that adoption workers will not let her talk to prospective parents, because she is "too realistic."

In 1993 Karyn S. adopted a beautiful little girl, the third generation in her birth family to be removed from the birth parents because of alcohol and neglect. Karyn and her husband adopted their daughter twenty years after the famous article on FAS appeared in *The Lancet,* but were not warned of the possibility of alcohol damage and only learned about FASD through the activities of our Toronto support group. Prior to the adoption, Karyn's social worker advised her to read books by Lois Melina and the writing team of Judith Schaffer and Christina Lindstrom (all three are American). Although the 1998 version of Melina's *Raising Adopted Children* mentions the possibility of fetal alcohol damage, the author glosses over any possibility of long-term effects. Similarly, Shaffer and Lindstrom's *Ultimate Resource Book for Adoptive Families,* published in 1991, mentions FAS only briefly, and wrongly suggests that, "Research does not take into account the effects of a warm, nurturing environment on the child's capacities." Karyn's daughter has been diagnosed with ARND, and despite the family's best efforts, she's now an out-of-control adolescent.

Ann Streissguth's secondary disabilities study indicates that a "warm, nurturing environment," which most adoptive parents give their children, is not enough. Alcohol-affected children need to be diagnosed as soon as possible; the parents need to understand their children's often-invisible neurologic birth defects; and both parents and children need strong support from the community, especially the education system. Without these elements in place, children and families are at high risk of parent burnout and adoption breakdown.

Infancy

Some people say, "If you have a person with fetal alcohol, you do A, B and C," and I find that's dangerous because there's no one technique, and having a cookbook sets the stage for rigidity. A cookbook provides people with a prescription, a recipe for doing things. What I believe that the research is providing for all of us is a series of ingredients, and what we can then do is become our own informants and pick and choose among the ingredients to create a good fit with the individual.

—Diane Malbin, Family Empowerment Network
Conference, Ann Arbor, Michigan, November 2, 1999

Because each individual with fetal alcohol damage has experienced a slightly different kind of exposure, all children with FASD are a little different, even as newborns. In her book, *Fetal Alcohol Syndrome: A Guide for Families and Communities,* Ann Streissguth outlines conditions that babies with FASD may display in infancy: tremulousness, irritability, disrupted sleep/wake cycles, weak suckle and failure to thrive. Other possible physical complications may include heart defects, organ and skeletal malformations, cleft lips and palates, hip displacement, scoliosis, seizures, hearing and visual problems, inflammation of the middle ear and pneumonia.

Nan in Toronto, the adoptive mother of a young adult female, remembers her daughter at nine months as a baby prone to tantrums. When put in a playpen, for example, she'd go into a screaming rage and fling her bottle across the room. Nan says that the first time it happened, "Her fingers were in a fist, her face as red as a tomato, and she was screaming." Nan checked for bumps and bruises, but there was no indication of any kind of injury. This behaviour was the first of countless puzzling rages as her daughter grew to adulthood. Nan now believes that her daughter has struggled lifelong with invisible sensory integration problems and learning disabilities that could have resulted from prenatal alcohol exposure.

We don't know what Colette was like as a newborn, except that she made many trips to hospital for problems such as salmonella and severe diaper rash, probably related to parental neglect. Taken into care at the age of eight months, she was placed with inexperienced foster parents—and cried for the next month. She then went to live with the experienced Newbiggings, and "quickly settled in to become a happy and contented baby," meeting all the normal milestones, and walking alone at eleven months.

I now believe baby Colette was suffering from "stranger anxiety," which often sets in at about eight months, when babies realize that their mother is not there, and may cry desperately in panic until she returns. What must she have been feeling—torn from her mother at that age? It's possible that, for most of our transplanted children, attachment problems are a separate struggle, not caused by prenatal alcohol, but adding to its insult.

The Golden Age

I better enjoy their younger years while I can. You know, the screaming meltdowns, the into everything, the hurting each other, the no fear of strangers or heights, the diapers, the piles of wet bedding to wash every day, the looking at you with a blank look as they try to understand what you said as you try to say it

*several different ways to see if it will finally absorb in some
brain cell. The spilled juice, the scattered food, the liquid soap
smeared all over the entire bathroom, the rotting food hidden in
a corner under a dresser . . .*

—POST FROM CAROL PEAVEY, SPRAGUE,
WASHINGTON, ADOPTIVE MOTHER OF FIVE YOUNG CHILDREN
AND ONE YOUNG ADULT MALE, ALL WITH FASD.

Ann Streissguth and others have remarked that the preschool years are
often a "golden age" for children with FASD. Although Colette was
always big for her age, and many alcohol-affected children are tiny, she
otherwise fit the description of the "golden" preschooler with FASD:
physically beautiful, bright-eyed, inquisitive, generally delightful and
quick to learn hands-on. But many preschool children with FASD are
already beginning to collect various psychiatric diagnoses, such as
attention deficit hyperactivity disorder (ADHD), oppositional defiant
disorder (ODD) and reactive attachment disorder (RAD). Therapists
who attempt to treat children with these diagnoses without understanding the underlying neurological damage of FASD are generally
not successful.

Chris Margetson of Guelph, Ontario, says that as an infant her biological son, Joe, with FAS, was a difficult eater and sleeper. He sat up
late and didn't walk until nearly three, but even before he was walking
"he would crawl out of his crib and find his way into the kitchen." Chris
would discover the pint-sized Houdini sitting on top of the stove, surrounded by the peanut butter and crackers he had somehow managed
to find. "I had to put a lock on the outside of his bedroom door, even
though I knew it was not safe, because it was more unsafe to not do it."

Chris got Joe into day care when he was about three, and then, she
says, "The phone calls started." She frequently had to leave work as a
result of Joe's behaviour. On one occasion, he stabbed his seat-mate
with scissors; on another, he ran head-first into a brick wall while looking through a magnifying glass! After that episode he required stitches.

The Fearless Factor

Colette's non-identifying information describes her as "an active inquisitive child" who at eighteen months was "climbing stairs with no fear . . . always getting into dangerous situations." The fearlessness of many children with FASD fills their parents with both pride and terror. Sue Truax of South Dakota is the adoptive mother of Eldon, of Sioux heritage, who began seeing a counsellor at two and a half. "He originally started because he was afraid of things he shouldn't be: bugs, rain, toy cars. He was not afraid of things he should be: climbing to the roof of my house, running into the street, playing with fire." Seven years of therapy—cognitive learning, anger management and play therapy—have helped greatly.

One morning I looked out of my second-story office to see five-year-old Colette waving at me—from a giant beech tree in the backyard. Judy Pakozdy of Whitehorse, Yukon, saw her son Matt's red sweater apparently caught in the branches at the top of a forty-foot pine tree—and then realized he was still wearing it. Other preschoolers with FASD have climbed trellises, basketball standards and streetlight poles. Toronto's Kim Meawasige tells of the terrifying Hallowe'en when, at dusk, she discovered two-year-old Brenda, naked except for a fuzzy rainbow clown wig, hanging by one hand from a TV antenna, thirty feet up, gaily waving at passersby.

In his book about children with FASD, *Watch for the Rainbows*, co-authored with Frances M. Kapp, the neuropsychiatrist Dr. Kieran O'Malley writes, "They will attempt physical feats that commonly intimidate many children their own ages." He notes that this behaviour is often labelled as "severe ADHD (attention deficit hyperactivity disorder):"

> The overzealous use of medication to socially control this natural exuberance is not always the most appropriate intervention. Instead, we should be able to acknowledge that children with FASD are not often encumbered by the same fears as other children, and if possible

we can let them enter their wild, physical world of excitement and unpredictability.[29]

Vulnerability to Predators

The confidence and fearlessness of many alcohol-affected children can make them extremely vulnerable to predatory children and adults. Carol Peavey, of rural Washington, wrote of a family reunion, distraught that relatives thought it was "wonderful" that her five children with FASD, aged three to nine, "would go to anyone and sit on their laps"—even people they had never met before. Once, when a truck pulled into their yard, her children ran up to it before the truckers even got out, excitedly asking them questions. Charlie, six at the time, explained to his mom that the men told them their names, so they weren't strangers.

In our family, Cleo would anxiously cling to Brian or me in any new situation, or when strangers arrived. Colette, on the other hand, was supremely confident, and we were proud of her, unaware that her fearlessness was related to an inability to predict consequences, and could have had tragic results.

Potty Problems

The FASlink archives list more than two hundred posts from parents discussing the toilet-training problem, and more than thirty about bed-wetting (enuresis). When Anne Marie was four, Claudia attended a class at The Arc (an organization that works with adults and children with intellectual disabilities) on toilet-training, and was told that the little girl should have her feet flat on the floor and be stabilized on all three sides. "I wedged a very small potty in between the toilet and the bathtub, close to the wall. It worked."

My theory is that many children with FASD may be delayed in learning to interpret the message from the bladder, and in some cases, the bowels as well. At night, many are very deep sleepers, and again, the message fails to come through. If Brian and I had realized that Colette's frequent daytime "accidents" (until the age of ten) were a neurological problem and not the result of carelessness, we would have spared her much nagging and humiliation.

School Age

These children are "stimulus-bound," and so their innate extro-version and exuberance can become magnified in a high-stimuli environment—for example, a classroom with a lot of noise or visually distracting images. So the common classroom that nur-tures richness in the environment as a method of enhancing learning is probably the worst type of environment for children with FASD.

—Dr. Kieran D. O'Malley, neuropsychiatrist,
Watch for the Rainbows

Donna Debolt talks of the increasing gap between our expectations of children with FASD and their performance. Even though many alcohol-affected children have low-normal to normal IQs, they gener-ally perform at about two-thirds of their chronological age. If a two-year-old performs at the level of an eighteen-month-old, few people will notice. When a six-year-old seems more like a four-year-old, teachers will begin to show concern. When a twelve-year-old has the academic skills of an eight-year-old, the schools often just throw up their hands.

Even in kindergarten, Anne Marie was told, "If you don't finish your work, you don't get recess." She had no recess until Claudia asked the teacher to send the work home. When the school psychologist insisted that Anne Marie needed Ritalin, Claudia explained that Anne Marie is not classically hyperactive. "She's not very physically wild, but she can lose her train of thought, and someone has to bring her back to it." Anne Marie's pediatric psychiatrist wrote a note indicating that Ritalin was not appropriate. The teacher, unconvinced, responded by offering to find Claudia, "a doctor who can make Ritalin work." (Claudia turned down the offer.)

Dr. Kieran O'Malley, a neuropsychiatrist who works closely with Ann Streissguth at the University of Washington Fetal Alcohol and Drug Unit, told me that Ritalin often does not work in children with FASD, and may make them even more restless or aggressive. He says that preliminary research indicates that Dexedrine is a better "first line psychostimulant" for alcohol-affected children. Currently, many FASlink parents are hoping that a new medication, Strattera, will help their children with attention deficits.

The school's lack of understanding of Anne Marie's invisible disabilities is typical. Last time I checked the FASlink archives, there were 1,365 posts from parents requesting advice on how best to handle an IEP (individual education plan) meeting—or reporting on frustrating meetings with teachers. (IEPs are sometimes known by different initials.)

> I went to the IEP meeting with our attorney and the psychologist who does social skills training and behaviour plans, and still got no place. The school absolutely refused to acknowledge any medical diagnoses made by any doctor! They said the diagnoses were too old! I said that FAS, microcephaly, cerebral palsy, etc. do not go away—they are lifelong problems. . . . They also said that as one diagnosis said FAS and another said FAE, they are contradicting each other and are both wrong. They refused to agree to follow the social skills and behaviour plan that our psychologist set up. . . . The lawyer says I can't fight it. (Joan Kaplan, New Jersey)

Lying, Stealing, Violence

When I asked FASlink correspondents what drove them craziest about their children with FASD, three behaviour problems came up over and over again: violence towards people, animals and property; stealing, otherwise known as "collecting" or "borrowing"; and lying, which Brian and I now call "creative reconstruction."

Colette was rarely violent as a child; however, in adolescence she kicked a hole in a wall, and on another occasion threw a hairbrush at a stained-glass window in our hall, cracking it. Gentle with animals, she fought only with her sister—and both girls always claimed the other had started it.

Many parents of children with diagnosed or undiagnosed FASD tell of frequent phone calls from teachers and discouraging school review meetings. I recall receiving only two phone calls in Colette's entire school career. When she was in fourth grade, a five-dollar bill went missing from a classmate's desk, and the evidence pointed to Colette—who was spending as wildly as Mack the Knife. The second call came when she was in eighth grade at private school, when she "borrowed" a miniature bottle of cognac from Brian's liquor cabinet, intending to share it with her classmates. She was suspended for three days. When Colette tells this story, the tiny airline bottle has become "a bar in my locker."

> For the most part, the majority of children with FASD do not intentionally lie. However, as caregivers well know, neither do they necessarily always tell the truth. The reasons behind this paradox are both various and complex. In many cases, the children simply are unable to fully distinguish reality from fantasy. . . . Almost all children will occasionally lie, at least temporarily, to protect themselves from punishment. Children with FASD, however, often display what could more aptly be described as, "creative thinking." Their attitude seems almost to be, "If I think it, it must be so."
>
> The issue of lying, or perceived lying, is the widespread reason that teachers feel the child with FASD is labelled as a troublemaker and as being untrustworthy. The perception of these children's lying becomes complicated by sustained memory problems, which are one of the unfortunately enduring legacies of prenatal alcohol exposure. (Dr. Kieran D. O'Malley, *Watch for the Rainbows*)

Desperately Seeking Support

The experiences of the Barkers and the Franks are not unique: countless neurologically damaged children are not receiving the help they need from schools or the community. Birth, adoptive and foster parents, desperately seeking answers and support from educators and social service workers, often find only ignorance, denial and a refusal to learn more.

Since Adam left the Frank home in 1998, he has been in a foster home, then back with his birth parents (briefly—his father had just been released from prison for murder, and his mother was still drinking), then into a group home. He is now in yet another foster home. Lynn has learned that his biological mother has been diagnosed with ARND, and all of his siblings have been removed from her care. As for Adam, he's one more stack attack victim, heading for trouble.

Lynn says that the adoption breakdown process left her "feeling hopeless and inadequate," worrying about the long-term impact on her whole family and her marriage. "When there is a death in the family, there are rituals and accepted ways of recognizing and supporting the grief and loss. But when an adoption breaks down there is nothing but a deep, dark abyss of despair—compounded by the condemnation of those who do not understand that all the love in the world cannot fix FASD."

What Could Have Helped

Both the Barker and the Frank families acquired their "transplanted" children in the early 1990s, nearly twenty years after fetal alcohol syndrome was officially defined. All of these children and their parents would have benefited from early diagnosis. They also needed real help, from informed doctors, psychiatrists, social workers and teachers who understood the many side effects of prenatal alcohol damage.

Adam was already showing signs of attachment problems when he was just two, and should never have been placed in a family with three demanding siblings, two of whom had family histories that indicated possible FASD. Lynn Frank is proud of her aboriginal heritage, and was delighted to be able to share her cultural knowledge and interest with her children. Adoption workers were equally pleased to place four native children in this home, without informing them of the possibility of fetal alcohol damage, and the resulting stress this could place on the family. All four of the Franks' adopted children should have been screened for FASD before adoption. As part of the pre-adoption process, the Franks deserved realistic information about possible prenatal alcohol damage in children available for adoption. This kind of training is now in place in Alberta and some other parts of North America.

Adam might have done better as an only child in a quiet household geared to his many needs, or in an experienced family with teenaged brothers or sisters. He also needed a community that understood his disabilities, and a physician knowledgable in medications that could have curbed his impulsiveness and frightening rages. "I will miss him all my life," Lynn recently wrote to me. "I still struggle with the grief of having to accept that all of our efforts with Adam were not enough. Until society and governments accept the reality of FASD and provide appropriate interventions and support, these kinds of tragedies will continue to devastate families."

Anne Marie Barker was lucky to have been placed in infancy with a bright, sensitive foster mother with school-age sons. The entire family quickly became committed to the little girl, and with no other preschoolers to care for, Claudia Barker had time and energy to deal with Anne Marie's complex neurological problems.

The Barkers hope that Anne Marie will be able to return to public school. The new principal and school trustees seem willing to explore methods of dealing with alcohol-affected children. Strategies have been developed by knowledgeable teachers and other professionals all around the world, but schools that offer special accommodation for these youngsters are rare. Winnipeg's David Livingstone School is unique. Its quiet, highly structured classrooms, designed for children with FASD, offer low pupil-teacher ratios, few distractions, much repetition and an enormous amount of gentle nurturing—exactly what Claudia Barker was able to do for her daughter at home.

CHAPTER TEN

"This Mask I Wear, Can You See Through It?"

The song she wrote was not a song
it was the way of her life,
written down in make-believe,
the way she wanted people to see her.

The song was tender and forgiving
was bright and full of sorrow,
she had always hid behind her long hair,
where no one could see her tears . . .

—JENNIFER WOODWARD, SIXTEEN, LIVING WITH FAS

In summer 1997, when seventeen-year-old Colette was wired on crack and living over the pool hall, I was thrilled to discover that a FASlink friend lived near our country cabin. Edith Woodward and her husband, Harold, had adopted their only child, Jennifer, when she was two and a half. Diagnosed with FAS at thirteen, Jennifer is only a year younger than Colette. Brian and I arranged to visit the Woodwards on our next trip to the cabin.

I naively hoped that Colette and Jennifer, close in age, sharing the same disability and both passionate about animals and the outdoors, might become friends. But on meeting Jennifer, I realized how unlikely that was; the two had little in common. Colette was a street-smart rogue sunflower, while slight, dark-haired Jennifer was shy and gentle, a fragile forest violet. Because she had been bullied and exploited by schoolmates and misunderstood by her teachers, Jennifer had been home-schooled by her mother since sixth grade. She showed us her fashion drawings—mostly ornate ball gowns—and read us some of her poetry. Protected by her loving parents in a small town where the only street is three blocks long, Jennifer reminded me of a fairy-tale princess—Sleeping Beauty or Rapunzel in blue jeans. In one of her poems, she wrote:

> *This mask I wear, can you see through it?*
> *Can you see I'm sad and my crown is too small to fit?*

The contrast between Jennifer and Colette illustrates the vast differences in the fetal alcohol spectrum. Each adolescent and young adult with FASD is as unique as a snowflake. Not all are delinquents: some give their families few problems, and lead relatively normal lives. For example, one young man of aboriginal heritage, now in his twenties, was diagnosed with prenatal alcohol damage as a preschooler; he graduated from a two-year program at community college, and recently married a fellow student, who was entranced by his solid, cheerful, generous personality and sense of humour. Recognizing his difficulty in handling money, his bride serves as his "external forebrain" where their budget is concerned.

A Lonely Child in an Adult's Body

What happens when an alcohol-affected thirteen-year-old has the emotional maturity and academic skills of a child of eight, the sizzling hormones of an adolescent, and, if female, possibly the physical maturity of a twenty-year-old? He or she is likely to become a pariah in school just when it seems most important to be popular. Often misunderstood by peers and the community since early childhood, adolescents with FASD are likely to have emotional problems. Jennifer Woodward suffers from depression and has been on anti-depressants since she was thirteen. Many adolescents with FASD "solve" their problems by self-medicating with alcohol or street drugs—as Colette did. Since 1997, I have learned that our daughter's undiagnosed primary and secondary disabilities are classic characteristics of FASD. Classic, too—unfortunately—is the lack of awareness of the fetal alcohol spectrum by many teachers, therapists and other professionals.

> Twenty years ago I was thrilled to bring home my infant daughter. In a letter to her birth mother I stated, "you gave her the gift of life, and I promise to help her make the most of it."
>
> I have failed dismally. Had anyone intimated to me then what life held in store for us, I would have totally dismissed them, not merely disbelieving, but self-righteously knowing that my mothering, my love, my total commitment would endow my child with happiness, health, self-esteem, self-worth, knowledge, experience and fulfilment. I could not have been further from the truth. Indeed, my daughter has garnered knowledge and experience I hope never to have, not even in my wildest nightmares. I have learned the hard way a harsh lesson: love is not enough. Mothering my daughter has been the most humbling experience of my life. (Mary Horner, Nelson, British Columbia, mother of daughter with FASD)

Puberty is difficult enough for ordinary youngsters, but when a child is living with the neurological impairment of prenatal alcohol, it can be catastrophic. On OlderFAS, a listserv for parents of adolescents and young adults with prenatal alcohol damage, one mother wondered if other adolescent females with FASD also "put themselves down as no-good and worthless, even walk in a posture of extreme defeat?"

"When girls hit puberty, their whole social landscape seems to change," Professor Robert Schacht of Northern Arizona University responded, referring to Carol Gilligan's book, *In a Different Voice.* In their desire to be popular, many young women begin comparing themselves with other females, and become depressed by their own seeming flaws. But when the young woman has FASD, "There's a double whammy: at just the age when peer relations become more important, social cueing gets more subtle and abstract. Our young women realize on some level that they're not able to keep up socially, and that adds to their depressed mood." Recently, when going through Colette's old school materials, I found a note she had written to herself at fifteen, while living at Hincks Farm and attending the local high school.

> Today Something strange happened! It's not because I've got the Flu. But when I'm by myself I find that I just brake down and start crying. I've woken up crying on nurmous occasions a bunch of times. This has happen at the Farm and only about twice has it happened at home! Personly, I think I'm suffering from a Depression or I'm just weird!

Surrounded by counsellors and psychiatrists, she nevertheless kept her feelings to herself. Certainly, this note would have set off alarm bells for staff, Brian and me, if any of us had seen it.

Young men with FASD seem equally susceptible to the double whammy of failed social cues. Generally unable to succeed in the classroom or in an entry-level job, they may find TV far easier. Watching sexy videos, commercials for beer and fast cars, and wrestling and cop shows, they begin looking for the glitz of TV in the real world. Often, they drift away from school and into alcohol and drugs, gangs, crime—and similarly damaged sexual partners.

Alcohol-affected young men and women can magically zero in on each other in the largest crowd by a sexual sixth sense that the FASD advocate Mary Horner calls "electro-alcoholic attraction." The daughters of OlderFAS correspondents tend to have similar boyfriends: drop-outs, drifters, drug users, dealers and petty criminals. These young males are often emotionally or physically abusive: many seem to be "stack attack" victims. These young people can give each other affection, physical gratification, companionship, comfort and a degree of acceptance they may rarely have encountered before.

In her book *Fetal Alcohol Syndrome: A Guide for Families and Communities,* Ann Streissguth describes the behavioural characteristics of individuals with FASD. After interviewing hundreds of parents and caregivers of alcohol-affected children and adults, she and fellow researchers noted thirty-six items on the "Fetal Alcohol Behavior Scale." Six key characteristics are related to a disability in "modulating incoming stimuli,"—a problem known as *"poor habituation."* Individuals with FASD may

- become overstimulated in social situations or crowded rooms
- over-react
- display rapid mood swings set off by seemingly small events
- have poor attention spans
- have difficulty completing tasks
- misplace things.

Irish researcher Dr. Jennifer Little has discovered that a five-month fetus of a woman who drinks lightly may also display poor habituation, and this condition persists in infancy: see chapter 5. Five other key characteristics of alcohol-affected children and adults are related to their poor cause-and-effect reasoning, especially in social situations. They often alienate friends and family because they

- seem unaware of the social consequences of their behaviour
- show poor judgement in whom to trust
- interrupt with poor timing
- can't take a hint and need strong clear commands
- love to be the centre of attention.

Streissguth notes that not all of the above items apply to every person with FASD, and these common characteristics are not meant to replace a diagnostic examination.[30]

Cast Adrift in a Knowledge-Based Society

Adolescents who fit Streissguth's behavioural profile have difficulty endearing themselves to parents, peers and teachers. Educators currently have many other problems on their minds: in most of North America, school boards are underfunded and school staffs are overworked and burdened by paperwork. Why should teachers and principals feel sympathetic towards adolescents who don't complete assignments, fail to pay attention and may be disruptive in class—if they bother to show up at all?

Teachers who take the trouble to inform themselves about FASD may be ignored or patronized. When Allan Mountford, an Ontario special education teacher, submitted a proposal for a region-wide program for alcohol-affected adolescents, including a training component on FASD for teachers, it was returned with the red-inked comment from an administrator: "This seems to be too much effort for too little return." This administrator seemed unaware that the "little return" could be fewer stressed teachers, fewer school dropouts, less crime and fewer unmarried teen pregnancies. In his self-published book, *'Cause It's Not My Fault,* based on his M.Ed. thesis, Mountford outlines the difficulties of the adolescent with FASD:

> They have trouble with change. Simple things like breakfast being two minutes early or a school bus arriving three minutes late can have a devastating result over the entire day. To consider the number of changes a student experiences in a day (e.g. subject changes, seating changes, teacher changes . . .) is to understand the stresses that some of these adolescents must endure.

Other invisible stresses of junior and senior high school include the labyrinth of hallways, the increasingly abstract nature of academic subjects, the clanging of bells, hallway chaos and noise between periods, the difficulty of remembering locker combinations, and the fact that high school students are expected to not act like "little kids." Mountford adds that teenagers with FASD deal with stress in numerous ways: from anxiety, frustration and shut-down to major mental health issues such as depression, aggression, abuse of alcohol and drugs or suicide. Noting that students with FASD are more likely to complete school if they have high-quality advocates, he recommends that each student be assigned one long-term advocate (the "external forebrain" again) throughout junior and senior high school.

I've observed that the alcohol-affected students who seem to do best are those in small, self-contained classrooms. Colette did well in such programs, and if she had been able to attend the same classroom throughout high school, she might have graduated. In the Waldorf system of private schools founded by Rudolph Steiner of Germany in 1919, the children's teacher moves with them from grades one to eight, and the children are taught in a hands-on, concrete way. In the Waldorf high school (part of the larger school), classes are small, usually one class per academic year, with no more than twenty-eight students, and each class is assigned a teacher-advisor who moves with them through high school.

Public school systems often ignore the fact that most learning-disabled children have great problems with change, and tend to do best in a small classroom. Many school boards believe that if a child succeeds in the self-contained classroom, it's time to move him or her back into the mainstream. It's ironic that the students succeeding in the small classrooms often have much lower IQs than the teenagers at the "high-functioning" end of the FAS spectrum—who are sinking like stones in the regular classroom.

Suspending kids is crack cocaine for teachers: it's addictive! (Jo Nanson)

Ann Streissguth's secondary disabilities study indicates that more than 70 percent of alcohol-affected males between twelve and twenty are likely to have a history of "disrupted school experience," characterized by suspension, expulsion or dropping out. The study found that 30 percent of females with FAS and 50 percent of females with ARND in this age group also had disrupted school attendance.[31]

Suspending an acting-out adolescent merely rewards him for inappropriate behaviour, while also putting him even further behind academically. The people who get punished are the parents, who worry about what mischief their child is going to get into during those empty "holidays." Assigning the student to lunchtime or after-school chores—scrubbing washrooms, picking up schoolyard trash, tidying the school library or some other kind of useful school-community service—could strengthen the student's fragile connection with the school and even be enjoyable.

> Sitting there in school, it was just like the teacher's words were buzzing around outside my head. (Colette, describing high school)

Almost every secondary school teacher has worked with adolescents with undiagnosed FASD—often wondering why these perplexing young people behave as they do. The Streissguth study indicates that among alcohol-affected students with disrupted school experience, about 70 percent have attention problems and 60 percent repeatedly failed to complete schoolwork. Nearly half had failed a grade in school. The most frequent behaviour problems were difficulties in getting along with peers (60 percent), repeatedly being disruptive (60 percent), talking back to teachers (45 percent) and fighting and truancy (38 percent).[32]

Parents of such students often feel they are being blamed by the school: why can't Mom or Dad *make* this kid shape up? Many parents attempt to solve the truancy problem (as I did) by driving their child to school; the youth goes in the front door of the school and sneaks out the back. Most high schools do not phone parents of truant students, so parents may not even be aware of skipped classes until report cards are mailed.

Most parents of adolescents with learning problems are justifiably worried that their children will be cast adrift in today's knowledge-intensive society. Many of us mortgage our homes and our future security to send the youngsters to a private school offering small classes and lots of structure. Some teenagers do well in such an environment, particularly if the school understands the learning problems resulting from prenatal alcohol damage. If Colette had been able to continue through high school in Mr. Connolly's small, highly disciplined junior high classroom at Montcrest, she might have graduated. But even expensive private schools can fail: the misbehaviour and truancy of the alcohol-affected adolescent may continue. My friend Nan and her husband invested more than $21,000 to send their fifteen-year-old daughter with probable FASD to boarding school. She lasted six months before being expelled for missing curfew, alienating fellow students by her thoughtless behaviour, writing slanderous letters to classmates and failing to do any schoolwork at all.

Even more frightening is the story told to me by the adoptive mother of seventeen-year-old "Shaun." Diagnosed with learning disabilities and ADHD, with an emotional age of around eleven, Shaun has a family history and behaviour that strongly indicate undiagnosed FASD. In his second year at an expensive military-style private school a three-hour drive from home, he lost all interest in learning. Finally, the fed-up principal told the young man he was free to leave, and walked him to the gates of the school, stranding him without money. The parents were not informed until the following day, and were terrified for his safety until he phoned home three days later, asking to be picked up from a friend's home in a nearby city. Back home, he decided to return to school. But would the principal have stranded an *eleven-year-old* so far from home? Shaun's learning and behaviour problems put him at risk of vanishing permanently.

A Too-Early Spring

When my daughter was about thirteen, I found her in bed with a boy. I had been home, but my daughter let him in the window. It was time for Depo Provera. We were at the doctor's office getting the shot, and she wanted to know if she would still get a balloon or sticker.

—FIONNA RAMIREZ, PASADENA, CALIFORNIA

Young people of both sexes with FASD are at high risk of being victimized sexually. Some of the alcohol-affected women I interviewed for this book disclosed painful memories of being assaulted as children or adolescents, by family members or friends. A number of parents also confided that their children with FASD—ranging from school-age children to adults—had been sexually assaulted by persons in positions of trust or power. Alcohol-affected children and adolescents with FASD, low in self-esteem and desperate to be liked, are vulnerable to sexual predators—particularly if this person is a family member.

As well, girls with FASD often mature physically earlier than the norm, and many young alcohol-affected females delight in their precocious curves: they can't do math, but they *can* attract older men. The mother of one eleven-year-old daughter was shocked by her child's sexually enticing behaviour, prancing half-clad around her adoptive father. In Canada and Hawaii, fourteen is the legal age of sexual consent, even for children whose neurological disabilities mean that they are emotionally nine years old. This means that an adult cannot be prosecuted for seducing a teenager half his or her age, unless the adolescent is willing to claim that he or she was assaulted. In the rest of the United States, laws vary from state to state: generally, age of consent is between sixteen and eighteen.

In many areas, doctors will not put adolescent females on birth control without explaining what it's for. Lynn Frank's adolescent daughter Marie has full FAS, an IQ of 79, and is physically mature. Although she does well in English and reading, emotionally and socially she is about three years old. Afraid that her sweet and naive little girl might be sexually victimized, Lynn nevertheless does not want her to know that she's on birth control to prevent pregnancy:

> Because of the nature of FAS and these youngsters' inability to understand abstract concepts, telling them "You shouldn't have sex until you have a long-term meaningful relationship" isn't going to work. That long-term meaningful relationship could be five minutes long. Or the guy could promise her, "I'll have a long term meaningful rela-

tionship with you, as long as you do this with me." So you've got to make it a pretty concrete, black-and-white message: no sex till you're married.

A Tangled Knot of Disabilities

Streissguth's secondary disabilities study neatly outlines the problems that almost inevitably occur when young people with fetal alcohol damage are not diagnosed early, are misunderstood by family and school and fail to receive adequate support by the community. A tangled knot of connected problems often results. They are at high risk for a comprehensive list of problems, including addiction to drugs and alcohol; contact with the judicial system; incarceration for crime, mental illness or substance abuse; inappropriate sexual behaviour; problems with employment; and, unfortunately, repetition of their biological parents' histories of inadequate parenting. Those who are not diagnosed are at far greater risk. And whether they have been diagnosed or not, *almost 100 percent of individuals with FASD will be diagnosed with a mental health disorder during their lifetimes.* Sixty percent of adolescents with FASD will be diagnosed with attention deficit problems; about 40 percent with depression; almost 25 percent will have panic attacks; 20 percent will hear voices or see visions. About a quarter of young people with FASD will make suicide threats, and more than 10 percent will actually attempt suicide.

> Children and adolescents with FAS/ARND present problems of a Dual Diagnosis nature, e.g., organic brain dysfunction due to prenatal exposure to alcohol, and mental disorders (of a primary or secondary nature). These patients may as well present a true Triple Diagnosis clinical picture, especially in adolescence and young adulthood. Here we may see a combination of organic brain dysfunction, secondary mental health problems and co-morbid addiction problems. (Dr. Kieran D. O'Malley, at the Calgary FAS Conference, May 1999)

When Parents Can No Longer Cope

Many parents of adolescents with FASD find they can no longer have their children at home. When a teenager seems to have no conscience, uses drugs or alcohol, is violent with his siblings and refuses to go to school or get a job, even the most devoted parent finds herself in an "It's him or me" situation. Even after I knew in my gut that Colette's behaviour was the result of prenatal damage, and something she couldn't control, in August 1997 I *still* told her she couldn't live with us any longer, and drove her to a shelter. During the six months when she slept in a series of flophouses or in a park, we sometimes didn't hear from her for a week or more. At those times I feared the worst and became overwhelmed with guilt: I was the one who had made her leave, unable to stand the stress of her lies, stealing, rages and druggie behaviour.

Many parents of alcohol-affected adolescents eventually run out of emotional resources. Therapists may tell us that family stress is causing our child to misbehave, but they have it backwards: our adolescent's impossible behaviour is devastating the entire family. Wealthy families often send these children to boarding school. Others ask their local child protection agency to put the child in foster care or a group home—often the first step to the child's winding up on the street.

Group Home Disasters

Colette looks back on her eighteen months at the Hincks "Farm" with affection and nostalgia, but not all group homes have the warmth, combined with structure and supervision, that she enjoyed at Hincks. In working with other parents, I've observed that the staff in most group homes tends to be poorly educated and trained. Many of these residences believe that the youngsters in their charge must "learn to be responsible" by having the freedom to make mistakes. This philosophy is extremely dangerous to an alcohol-affected child operating at two-thirds his chronological age. George and Andrea are an Ontario couple whose daugher Sophie's ARND made her too difficult for them to cope with: the lies, stealing and truancy had become too much by the time she was fourteen. The local Children's Aid Society became involved, and she was placed in a coeducational youth treatment centre with a school on the premises. The parents were horrified to discover that because there was no supervision at night, she was meeting her boyfriend in the hallway after midnight—and who knows what was going on?

The parents complained, explaining that an adolescent with fetal alcohol damage requires full-time supervision (that "external forebrain"). The group home manager replied that, despite Sophie's diagnosis of ARND, she needed to take responsibility for her actions.

The parents later learned that during those midnight forays, Sophie had become pregnant, and the group home had arranged an abortion for her, without informing them. By Canadian law, at fourteen, she can be sexually active with whomever she chooses, and medical professionals are not required to inform parents, even if the youngster in question is emotionally nine years old. "Graduating" from the group home, Sophie moved in with a different boyfriend, and at seventeen gave birth to a baby, who was removed by child protection authorities.

Many children in group homes have been injured or killed. One homicide occurred within a two-hour drive of my home, when thirteen-year-old William Edgar was suffocated by a group home worker in Cavan, near Peterborough, in March 1999, while under the care of the local CAS. His mother suffers from schizophrenia, and both parents were alcoholics. William had the developmental delays, small size, visual problems, low-set ears and flat philtrum of full FAS. Prone to rages, illiterate, diagnosed with ADHD, mentally about six years old, he also had grey eyes, dimples and his own kind of mischievous smarts.

A photo in the *National Post* shows William, a Harry Potter lookalike with large round glasses and an impish grin, looking about nine. The youngster had been sat on, held face down on the floor for forty minutes by a child-care worker, because he refused to sit still on a chair as part of "sit" punishment for talking back. According to an article in Toronto's *Globe and Mail,* the worker did not notice anything wrong, and told another worker the boy was pretending to be asleep. The inquest jury learned that eleven children in this group home had been injured by staff, and seven had complained that they were unable to breathe when this method of "restraint" was used. A year before William's death, another boy in this group home had lost consciousness while restrained, and could not be revived for five minutes. Since 2001, several other North American adolescents with family histories and learning disabilities consistent with FASD have died while being "treated" for acting-out behaviour.

Set Up to Fail

To whom it may concern:

I am a student at Central Commerce High school and I'm looking for a part-time job mucking stalls or looking after hounds. I am experienced in both fields. I have been riding since I was two years old and I have grown up with dogs and have just acquired a hound myself.

I have worked at a breeding farm called Toft Hill Farms who breed Hanavarians [sic]. I also love animals and would go to the ends of the earth to get a job working with them . . .

—COLETTE'S LETTER TO PROSPECTIVE
EMPLOYERS, WRITTEN AT AGE SIXTEEN

Physically strong and a willing worker, Colette is typical of young people with FASD looking for employment in a job market where knowledge counts for more than muscle. As adults over the age of twenty-one, 79 percent of those studied by the Streissguth team had great difficulty finding work. The researchers defined job success as supporting oneself with employment; earning $280 a week or more (in 1996 U.S. dollars); or working at least half time and having had no more than three jobs in the past two years. Researchers listed many problems that employees with FASD have on the job: a low frustration threshold, poor task comprehension, poor judgment, social problems, unreliability, difficulties in managing anger, problems with supervision and lying. My online correspondents indicate that stealing is another frequent cause of being fired. The Streissguth researchers found that no alcohol-affected adults with IQs of less than 70 were able to succeed on the job. The single most protective factor was a driver's licence, "followed by never experiencing violence, an early diagnosis, and living in a nurturing and stable home for over 72 percent of life."

The statistics don't reflect the pain felt by alcohol-affected young people as they repeatedly lose their jobs. At eighteen, Colette was hired at an upscale burger restaurant. One hour before the place opened, she prepared tomatoes, dill pickles and lettuce. Then, "dressing" hamburgers, she had to cheerfully belt out songs with fellow workers, while remembering customers' choices: would they like mayo, mustard, ketchup, pickles, cheese, tomatoes, lettuce, hot peppers and/or alfalfa sprouts? After spending eight hours trying to multi-task and focus in a noisy, clattering environment, her face would be grey with exhaustion. After one month, she phoned in tears, telling me she had just been fired. When I picked her up, she was slumped miserably on a bench outside the restaurant, reminding me of the six-year-old who had so much difficulty learning to read. "I don't understand, Mom, I tried so hard," she sobbed.

Keeping focused in a full-time job is difficult for most alcohol-affected individuals. But I believe that she and many other people with FASD could succeed in part-time positions, providing that their basic needs were subsidized by government, and their employers understood their disabilities. The extra money they earned would be ploughed right back into the Canadian economy—mostly for food and clothing for themselves and their children.

Babies Having Babies

Dear Dad,

Well, I know you are very unhappy with my decision to have a baby, but I am serious about this. I understand it isn't like going out and getting a hamstear [hamster]. I think I've been really responsible about it. First of all, when I missed my period I went Right away to get a Blood test taken. Then when I found out it was positive I went to see Dr. B . . . who told me what kind of Vitamins to take and I got more Blood tests done to make sure I don't have anything that can effect the baby . . .

I bought the prenatal vitamins and are taking them Regularly. I'm Eating well, and on top of it I asked mom to buy me a Book Called "what to expect when Expecting" it's the pregnent woman's bible, it's a great book . . .

I Really want my Baby to have both grandparents around. I hope you can furgive me but I'm going through with it. I'm sorry if I hurt you but I really am serious about this I hope you understand that . . . I guess you don't want a kid who hasen't finished high school, and is pregnent, I guess you don't want another sasitic [statistic] For a daughter but Please don't Forget that you're my dad and I love you a lot, and I've always looked up at you and I would love my child to have a grandfather who can teach him/her how to Bake and to Love nature, and to work with wood, I want my kid to have the grand-Father I never had . . .

Love forever and always,
your daughter
Colette
(DATED APRIL 21, 1999)

That year, it seemed as if every mother of a young woman with FASD was dealing with her daughter's pregnancy, both in our Toronto support group and online. Not one of the young women was married, or over the age of twenty-one. Two were only sixteen. One nineteen-year-old was pregnant with her second child. Most of these grandmothers-to-be looked on anxiously as their daughters partied throughout pregnancy, seemingly not caring about the possible damage to the babies they were carrying.

Following the birth of their grandchildren, the new grandmothers began scanning and sending baby photos online—terrified that their beloved grandchildren might be damaged too. Were the wide-spaced eyes, cute little noses, and odd-shaped ears merely genetic, or were they caused by prenatal alcohol? As the infants grew older, we measured their progress against published "normal" milestones. We know that school will be the real test. Will our grandchildren struggle with the same learning difficulties, and the lack of understanding by the school system that so damaged their mothers? Do we have the energy to be advocates for yet another generation?

Shortly before her twentieth birthday, Colette gave birth to a seven-pound boy, fathered by her partner of two years. She had treated her pregnancy with the obsessiveness she had formerly attached to heavy metal music and drugs. Her TV viewing consisted mainly of parenting and baby shows, and her "bible" on pregnancy was dog-eared from reading and re-reading. She did not drink or use drugs, and we were amazed that the tomboy who never played with dolls was such a responsible, gentle mother.

Eighteen months later she gave birth to a baby girl, six weeks prematurely. Like her first pregnancy, this one was an "accident," and although Brian and I encouraged her to consider an abortion, Colette could not bring herself to do so. My sense is that for adopted children, who grow up without anyone who is truly "their blood," a genetic relative is a treasure. As Colette tenderly held her newborn daughter, as tiny as a kitten, hooked up to tubes in the neonatal intensive care unit, I remembered the seven-year-old who had helped to birth a calf, the twelve-year-old who had stayed up three nights with newborn puppies to make sure they would survive. She was a devoted mother to her babies—but now that they have developed strong personalities as preschoolers, she's finding parenting an almost impossible challenge.

All too often, children of mothers with FASD are shunted back and forth from extended family members to child protection agencies, and may even appear in tragic headlines. We know numerous grandparents who are raising their children's alcohol-affected children, and wondering how they will cope as senior citizens parenting difficult teenagers. Currently, there seems to be no appropriate contraceptive for young women who can't remember to take the Pill or change their contraceptive patch, hate the quarterly injections of Depo Provera, fear the invasiveness of Norplant (inserted into the upper arm) and find the notion of IUDs "yucky." Most of us encourage our children to become sterilized, but know this is unlikely to happen. Ann Streissguth told me of doctors actually *discouraging* young alcohol-affected women from having tubal ligations, even after they have had two or more children.

Many parents who have raised children with FASD—and I'm among them—view repeated and unplanned childbirth as cruel and unusual punishment to both the alcohol-affected mother and her resulting infants. The fertility of our children is frightening, particularly if they are continuing the patterns of their biological mothers— drinking or using drugs.

Many of us can look back on the family histories of our adopted children and add up the expense to the taxpayers of those years of social services—the father and other male relatives frequently in trouble with the law, and sometimes in jail; the rest of the continually expanding family on lifelong social assistance. In Colette's biological family, both parents (separated) live on social services income, and one brother is in frequent contact with the criminal justice system. Including Colette, at that estimated $2 million cost to taxpayers per alcohol-affected individual per lifetime, we're looking at $8 million for one family right there.

Just Another Missing Kid

Running away can be a frightening experience—for both the child and the parents. Your child becomes vulnerable as soon as he or she leaves home—potentially falling victim to drugs, drinking, crime, sexual exploitation, child pornography, or child prostitution. In the face of this, many parents may feel guilty or depressed . . . or even paralyzed by fear . . . The first 48 hours following the runaway are the most important in locating the child. Many runaway children return home during this 48-hour period.

—The National Center for Missing and Exploited Children (U.S.) website, www.missingkids.org

In Canada, more than 50,000 runaway adolescents are reported every year, and on any given day there are about 1,400 runaway cases in the Canadian Police Information System. About 6 percent of the Canadian runaways are reported as having fetal alcohol syndrome, and 8 percent of these are of aboriginal background.[33] Given the low rates of diagnosis, and the fact that four times as many people have invisible ARND as have FAS, it's probable that a far larger number of runaways—30 percent or more—may be living with the effects of prenatal alcohol.

Characteristics of a Runaway

The profile of runaway teenagers is almost identical to that of adolescents with FASD. According to Canada's *Missing Children Annual Report,* issued by the RCMP Missing Children's Registry, the most common reason for running away is intolerable family conflict, which may include physical or sexual abuse. Most runaways "did not perform well in school, often finding school an uncomfortable and frustrating experience." Most runaways have gone no further than ninth grade, and were perceived by teachers as troublesome. They tend to be extremely unhappy and lonely, and they lack self-esteem. As well, they exhibit internal conflict, psychological problems, inadequate social skills and poor coping and communication skills. Because they have no means of support and no skills that would make them employable, most become "involved in the sex trade, drugs, panhandling and other delinquent activities."

Many youngsters with FASD are "runners." By the time Colette was fourteen, she would vanish for days on end. One tiny, naive eighteen-year-old with an emotional age of eight went to the movies with her social worker, vanished from the women's washroom, and was found several months later in a scruffy apartment with a group of addicts. I know two adoptive mothers who have been thrilled to receive collect phone calls from opposite ends of the continent, from runaway adolescent daughters with ARND who desperately needed an air ticket to come home.

The Mystery of Mistie Murray

On May 31, 1995, petite, hazel-eyed, sixteen-year-old Mistie Murray of Goderich, Ontario, told her family she was going to band practice. It was a warm spring evening; she set out, wearing a distinctive green jacket bearing her name and the crest of the Seaforth District High School Girls Marching Trumpet Band. She never returned. Her best friend later told her parents that there had not been a band practice that evening, and that instead she'd had a secret date.

Three months later, her loving adoptive father, Steve Murray, was arrested for allegedly throwing Mistie off his boat in the middle of Lake Huron, despite the lack of motive, opportunity or evidence. However, because Mistie was *adopted,* Goderich police were convinced that her father had a motive for murder. Although they dragged the lake throughout the summer of 1995 without finding her body, they chose to believe in homicide. Why else, they asked, would a young girl vanish without taking her belongings? If they knew about the impulsiveness and poor judgment of adolescents with FASD, they would not ask that question.

Mistie's mother was a troubled young woman living in an atmosphere of poverty and substance abuse, and her little girl was taken and placed in a therapeutic foster home when she was two. It was three years before social workers felt she was mentally healthy enough for adoption. When Anne and Steve Murray adopted her, she was five years old but weighed only thirty-two pounds, less than my two-year-old granddaughter. Her constant ear problems, small head, learning disabilities, poor social skills, behaviour problems as an adolescent and troubled birth family history point to a strong probability of prenatal alcohol damage.

Working closely with her lawyer, Brian Greenspan, Anne Murray researched complex information about the timing of the alleged murder, which proved that her husband could not possibly have been responsible for Mistie's disappearance. During the preliminary hearing, Greenspan discovered evidence, hidden by the police, of ninety-seven sightings of Mistie, many by people who knew her, in the year after she vanished. Most of these sightings were in the weeks after she disappeared.

Anne Murray knew that her husband was innocent, and her website, www.mistie.com, details numerous improprieties by Goderich police. They did not attempt a proper search for Mistie, and the national information they sent out described her as being five foot five and 125 pounds: two inches taller and fifteen pounds heavier than she really was. They ignored the ninety-seven sightings, which showed a trail from her home in Goderich to Clinton, London and Toronto, and did not report these sightings to the family or Child Find.

It took the jury only forty-five minutes to acquit Steve Murray, but the couple's marriage was shattered. "We're still friends," says Anne. "He spends most of his time on the road, driving transport trucks. We see each other every few weeks, but . . ." She gives a poignant shrug.

Because of Anne's efforts, a different police force was assigned to look into the Goderich investigation. The Murrays received a letter of apology from the Ontario Civilian Commission on Police Services, indicating that the Goderich Police Service had improperly investigated Mistie's disappearance due to insufficient staff, poor training and inadequate supervision.

During the summer of 2001, Anne received information that a young woman fitting Mistie's description had briefly stayed in a Vancouver shelter under the name "Mallory Lane." When asked if she was Mistie Murray, she fled. Police later showed Anne a photo of the young woman, but "the eyes and nose did not seem right: I don't think it was Mistie."

Anne has concluded that if Mistie is alive, she is incapable of choosing to be found. Needing closure to the tragedy that consumed their family for more than six years, Anne, Steve and their two adult sons held a Mass of Remembrance on November 10, 2001. "Turning Mistie over to God's hands," the Murrays said their goodbyes to the fragile little girl they had all loved so much, and will miss for the rest of their lives.

But what if Mistie had been diagnosed with fetal alcohol syndrome when she was young enough to be helped? A psychologist knowledgable in both FASD and attachment disorder might have helped the Murrays to give her the structure and boundaries she required. Even when Mistie "ran," a knowledgable police force would have understood that this is classic behaviour for alcohol-affected teens. Trained officers would have quickly followed up those leads from several classmates who saw her in nearby Clinton only days after she disappeared. Recognizing that a sixteen-year-old female with FASD has the emotions of a ten-year-old, will almost certainly take dangerous risks and is vulnerable to predators, they would have done everything in their power to find her alive.

No one will ever know whether police misjudgment resulted in the death of Mistie Murray. However, according to the U.S. National Center for Missing and Exploited Children, as soon an adolescent is reported missing, the search should begin—while the trail is still warm. Unfortunately, the "rights" of a sixteen-year-old, no matter what her emotional age, mean that she has the right to disappear, and police generally do not search actively unless foul play is indicated.

What Could Have Helped

Early diagnosis plus support for children with FASD in their younger years could have reduced some of the problems of the adolescents in this chapter. However, the normal high school, with its clatter, distractions and new independence, is not conducive to success for these youngsters.

Remember Teresa Kellerman's SCREAMS strategies? Just when adolescents most need supportive Structure, Cueing, Role Models, Environment, Attitude [ours], possibly Medication and Supervision, they are least likely to get it. As well, it's *normal* for teenagers to want to be independent, and to balk at controls, unless they have been trained from an early age to accept that they will always need that "external brain."

School administrators, staff and parents should go directly to "A" for Attitude, and understand that alcohol-affected adolescents may appear lazy or non-compliant, when in reality they are puzzled and miserable. In *'Cause It's Not My Fault,* Allan Mountford outlines strategies to help adolescents with diagnosed or suspected FASD succeed in school. Each student must be assessed for strengths and challenges. "If a teacher can determine how a student learns, the teaching style can be altered to contribute to success." Mountford cautions that many of these students have strong verbal skills but weak academic performance, and may experience a sudden drop in academic ability, because "the skills required for success in high school tend to be more analytical and abstract." He adds that when teens seem to have "wilful disregard for authority . . . [they] are in reality having problems translating verbal directions into action."

Every effort should be made to have youngsters with suspected FASD diagnosed, if this has not been already done. Teachers and administrators should be trained in how to deal with these youngsters, even if FASD is merely suspected, not confirmed. They will do best in small classes with hands-on work, such as in technical or co-op programs, and generally have great difficulty in math or foreign languages, often required for graduation.

Most teenagers with FASD require far more structure and supervision than normal adolescents, and more than many families can provide. When parents are burned out by their children's behaviour, social agencies usually offer foster care or a group home. Few agencies consider cheaper, less intrusive alternatives, such as paying for a part-time "mentor" (a college student, say) who could bring the youngster home from school, and "hang out" with him for a few hours each day, keeping him safe.

When modest part-time help is not enough, government spending on well-planned residential care could save millions of dollars in the long term by reducing the number of street kids surviving by their wits, and by crime. Almost every community in the industrialized world is desperately lacking in rehabilitation facilities for young adolescents with addiction problems. While protecting our citizens, investments of this kind would protect our damaged angels not only from themselves but also from evil predators who seek out the lonely and emotionally fragile.

CHAPTER ELEVEN

A Lifetime Sentence

*It was behind this school that the boy made his last sound, a
scream that carried through the night like a wildcat's. So pierc-
ing was his cry, it woke people living in a nearby house; they
peered out their windows into the darkness across the street.
There, they saw what must have looked like a group of people,
teenagers, dancing feverishly in a dark corner. They called the
police. It was 2:20 a.m.*

—JEFF GAILUS, *ALBERTA VIEWS*, MAY/JUNE 2001

When the cruiser pulled up to the school in Edmonton, Alberta, police
found four youths in the schoolyard, one of them covered in blood.
Then they found a fifth young man, slumped against the wall in a pool
of blood, unconscious, his battered face unrecognizable. He carried no
identification, but doctors found his name, Garrett Campiou, written
in ink on his thigh. Six feet tall, only fourteen years old, and of
aboriginal origin, he had been bounced through two sets of adoptive
parents and numerous foster parents. His biological and adoptive families had struggled with alcohol addiction, and a former foster mother
told Jeff Gailus that the youth suffered from fetal alcohol syndrome.

The little boy grew up in a series of broken homes, plagued by
poverty, neglect, accidental deaths and alcoholism. His adoptive parents

lived on welfare, and when Garrett was four his adoptive mother died in a car accident. His adoptive father, an alcoholic, was left to look after five children—and so began the little boy's journey through countless troubled homes: another stack attack victim.

On the night of the murder, Garrett told his adoptive father that he was going to visit his grandmother, a few blocks away. Instead, he wound up in the nearby schoolyard, drinking high-test malt liquor with four young men, two of whom beat him unconscious. Of native background as well, they shared similar family histories, and may also have had FASD.

Two weeks after the assault, doctors told the family that although Garrett's heart was still beating, his spirit had flown away. The people who loved him most burned ceremonial sweetgrass and prayed to the Creator. Then they gathered around Garrett, who was covered in bandages, and the doctor switched off the high-tech equipment that had kept his body alive.

Garrett is only one of the countless alcohol-affected youths and adults who die tragically every year, often at the hands of others. The impulsiveness and poor judgment of children with FASD can only be controlled through diagnosis and loving support. Those who grow up abused and neglected in a series of homes are at risk of the secondary disabilities: dropping out of school, addiction, unemployment, homelessness and trouble with the law. They may find themselves in situations of violence and brutality, and all too often someone else may find them dead.

The Prison of the Soul

We do not need one child born in this country with FAS. If we could get to the mothers . . . that would make a huge difference in crime rates.

—THE HONOURABLE ANNE McLELLAN, CANADIAN
MINISTER OF JUSTICE, SPEECH, OCTOBER 1999

New studies in neurology have discovered that what we call "conscience" resides in the brain, and may be linked to both the frontal lobes and the corpus callosum, two of the areas most sensitive to prenatal alcohol. With this knowledge, we as a society must begin to rethink the questions of good and evil, free choice and predetermination. For where, exactly, does the soul reside, if the choices you make are determined by your neurology?

When the Hon. Anne McLellan was federal Justice Minister, one of her departments, the Correctional Service of Canada, commissioned a report on FAS entitled *Fetal Alcohol Syndrome: Implications for Correctional Service,* published in 1998. The clear and concise study distills twenty-five years of international research on the relationship of FASD and crime into ninety-two double-spaced pages. The authors' simple recommendations could greatly help offenders with FASD, reduce recidivism and cut the costs of the criminal justice system not just in Canada, but throughout the world. The report's main suggestion is that authorities screen and assess arrested offenders who may have FASD, so that they can be given appropriate sentencing and programs. Unfortunately, few people involved in "corrections" seem to be paying any attention to this study.

The University of Washington secondary disabilities research indicates that about 60 percent of individuals with FASD will encounter "trouble with the law," and more than 40 percent will be incarcerated in a penal institution at some time in their lives. Males are at more risk than females, and worldwide statistics indicate that about four times as many man are incarcerated as women. People with FAE/pFAS/ARND, though brighter, are more likely to have encounters with the police than those with full FAS. Because they are invisibly damaged, they are seldom diagnosed or given adequate support. As well, their higher IQs mean that they are far more difficult for parents and the community to control.

About 40 percent of the crimes committed by participants in the Streissguth secondary disabilities study were crimes against persons: theft, shoplifting, burglary and assault. About a third of the participants committed their first offence between the ages of nine and fourteen, and this offence was most often shoplifting. Almost all committed their first offence before the age of twenty.

Youngsters with FASD tend to be incompetent shoplifters, often egged on by more skilful friends, who leave them holding the bag. Having a child arrested for shoplifting is a demeaning experience for a good parent—and some retail chains are now adding to family pain by sending threatening letters fining parents as much as $500 because a child pilfered an item as small as a tube of lipstick. Several American states and Canadian provinces have legislation that forces parents to pay for the crimes of their delinquent children.

Little Victims

Seventy-five percent of kids we see in our clinic have experienced physical abuse. We are not seeing fetal alcohol syndrome, folks— we are seeing fetal torture syndrome.

—Dr. Sterling Clarren, speech in
Whitehorse, Yukon, May 2002

The secondary disabilities study does not look at the statistics regarding the number of people with FASD who are *victims* of crimes. Every year, numerous children with FASD are injured or killed, some by persons who are also alcohol-affected, others by people in positions of trust, such as babysitters, caregivers or even parents. The words "fetal alcohol" are rarely used to describe these little victims and their families. Media articles may mention substance abuse and dysfunction, learning disabilities, attention deficit problems, attachment disorder or behaviour problems. But when parents or professionals familiar with FASD read about these cases, the case histories and symptoms are all too familiar.

Over the Easter weekend of 1999, residents of Calgary were horrified by the tragic deaths of four-year-old Derek Lynes with FAS, and his half-brother, three-year-old Phelan Layng, murdered early Good Friday morning by a vindictive babysitter. Phelan's mother, twenty-year-old Alanna Westergard, had entrusted her son and his half-brother to Robert Richard Cooper, a homeless twenty-two-year-old with a record of unemployment and drifting. Westergard had agreed to give him a place to stay in return for babysitting. Four-year-old Derek, whom she was raising as her own child, was the son of her ex-husband by his former girlfriend, a street person.

Westergard had gone to a party, and phoned home at 1:30 a.m. to say she was staying out all night. Furious with jealousy, Cooper put plastic bags over the children's heads and suffocated them. The children's mother returned home twelve hours later and was horrified to discover the children, tucked in their beds, stiff, purple, lifeless. At first, Cooper maintained that an unknown intruder must have killed them while he was asleep. He later sobbed out a rambling confession, and was charged with first-degree murder.

During the trial, the court heard that Cooper had described himself as having "two sides"—one kind and gentle, the other a "monster." According to the *Calgary Sun,* Cooper "showed no emotion" as he was sentenced to life imprisonment on two counts of second-degree murder. Cooper's history and lack of remorse indicate that, like tiny Derek Lynes, he may have been affected by alcohol before he was born.

Dangerous Liaisons

Prostitutes are at especially high risk of being victimized. Barbara Smith, FASD coordinator of the Victoria-based PEERS (Prostitutes Empowerment Education and Resource Society) says that her organization's research indicates that most sex trade workers have histories consistent with fetal alcohol damage. She cites a study by researchers Cecilia Benoit and Alison Millar that indicates that the majority of sex trade workers had been in foster care or group homes. This same research discovered that more than 90 percent of sex trade workers had been pregnant, averaging more than three times each, and only 25 percent of them had their children living with them. PEERS' research is consistent with the secondary disabilities study, in which 15 percent of interviewees reported promiscuous behaviour. The secondary disabilities study also indicates that about 70 percent of women with ARND will have alcohol or drug problems, which the PEERS researchers found to be an almost universal problem with sex trade workers, who are at high risk of bearing children with FASD.

"Ladies of the night" have always been in great danger of being injured or killed by their "clients." Canada's most horrific case is that of the more than fifty missing Vancouver prostitutes who disappeared during the 1990s and even earlier: nearly all were addicted to street drugs. On February 5, 2002, Vancouver police and the RCMP began an investigation on a pig farm in the suburb of Port Coquitlam, and arrested the owner, Robert William Pickton. Parts of the bodies of the missing women began to be found buried on the farm. As this book goes to press, the DNA of dozens of women has been identified at the site, along with enough forensic evidence to charge Pickton with twenty-two murders. The forensic investigation alone will cost more than $70 million.

Barbara Smith believes that most of the victims or suspected victims had prenatal alcohol damage. Photographs and histories on the website indicate that several were of aboriginal background and had alcoholic families; others were raised by foster or adoptive parents.

The stunningly beautiful Sarah DeVries, one of the missing women, was never diagnosed with fetal alcohol damage. But her story is achingly familiar to many adoptive parents of young females with FASD. Born in 1969, Sarah was adopted at eleven months by a university professor and a nurse, and raised in Vancouver's upscale Point Grey area. Of African-Canadian, aboriginal and Caucasian heritage, she was a happy, active little girl who, like Colette, loved horseback riding and was a fearless swimmer. Her adoptive mother, Pat DeVries, now has evidence that Sarah's birth mother may have been involved with the sex trade, alcohol and drugs as well.

In school, like many youngsters with FASD, Sarah had great difficulty with math. Maturing early, she was attracted to the dangerous Downtown Eastside, and by the time she was twelve had tried drugs, dropped out of school and got into trouble with the law. These learning and behaviour problems, as well as her tiny size (she was only five feet tall) and family history, are consistent with fetal alcohol damage. By twenty-two, Sarah, heavily into addiction and prostitution, had given birth to two children, who are being raised by her adoptive mother, Pat. Bright and delightful, her children have learning and attention-deficit problems, probably caused by Sarah's substance use in pregnancy. By the time her second child was born, Sarah was HIV-positive, but fortunately her baby was not affected.

Sarah vanished one night in April 1998, after telling her close friend Wayne Leng, "I'll call you." The last entry in her journal read: "I've been dead at least six times over in my heart. I should be six feet under. I truly believe I have a guardian angel watching my every move."

A Dearth of Research

Many of the behavioural features that are characteristic of children with FAS/FAE, such as attention deficits, hyperactivity, and impulsiveness, have been shown in longitudinal studies to be predictors of delinquency and adult criminal behaviour. Although there is substantial evidence suggesting a link between FAS and crime, there is a dearth of research examining FAS/FAE in the criminal justice system. In fact, there are no known studies reporting the prevalence of FAS/FAE in prisons.

—*Fetal Alcohol Syndrome: Implications for Correctional Service*, report by Correctional Service Canada, 1998

Although there is still little research regarding the prevalence of FASD in prison systems, one fascinating study looks at young offenders with

FASD. The report *Youth in the Criminal Justice System: Identifying FAS and Other Alcohol-Related Neurodevelopmental Disabilities,* was funded by the British Columbia government and written by Christine Loock, M.D.; Julianne Conry, Ph.D.; and Diane Fast, M.D., Ph.D. For one year, beginning on July 1, 1995, the team screened all youths remanded to the Inpatient Assessment Unit (IAU) of Youth Court Services in Burnaby, B.C. They point out that on any given day in the province, there are about 300,000 teenagers aged twelve to eighteen, and about 2 percent of them are in the criminal justice system, and one in one thousand is behind bars. The youths studied were 80 percent male, 20 percent female.

The report focused on 287 young offenders, aged twelve to eighteen, who had been remanded to IAU for psychiatric and psychological assessment. All had committed criminal offences, and most had pleaded guilty or been found guilty. Of the 287 young people, 224 (78 percent) were flagged for assessment for FASD, mainly on the basis of short palpebral fissure (eye slit length). Sixty-seven of them—23 percent—were eventually diagnosed with prenatal alcohol damage: four with FAS and sixty-three with pFAS or ARND. Several others displayed evidence of central nervous system damage, and might have been diagnosed with ARND if the researchers could have obtained family histories. Because many were not living with a biological parent, prenatal, birth and early developmental records and baby photographs were not always available.

All professionals involved in criminal justice should read this ground-breaking study, along with the book *Fetal Alcohol Syndrome and the Criminal Justice System,* written by two of the study's authors, Conry and Fast. One of the study's key findings was that the IQs of youth diagnosed with an "alcohol-related disorder" ranged from intellectually deficient to superior. Thirty-eight percent had an average IQ or higher. However, 62 percent had below-average intelligence, placing them "at greater risk of not understanding the consequences of their actions or fully comprehending the implications of court proceedings."

Like Ann Streissguth, the authors take pains to point out that many alcohol-affected people never become involved in the criminal justice system. Nevertheless, they state:

> The percentage of FAS in the youth remanded to IAU (4.5 percent) is 30 times the accepted world-wide incidence for this disorder. The percentage of youth with any alcohol-related diagnosis (23.3 percent) is 10 to 40 times the world-wide incidence. The data support the contention that this group is disproportionately represented in the juvenile justice system . . .

Julianne Conry, a psychologist, does not know if the rate of offenders with FASD—at least 23 percent in this assessment centre—is the same in other juvenile facilities or in the adult correctional system. "The rate could be higher or lower," she says. The Saskatchewan psychologist Jo Nanson says she believes that at least 25 percent of incarcerated inmates in that province have FASD, and the number is probably between 50 and 80 percent for inmates of low intelligence.

At press time, Corrections Canada is working with a research team led by Dr. Brian Grant and Dr. Ab Chudley to look at means of recognizing offenders with FASD. The researchers will develop and test a screening tool by assessing 100 inmates in a federal penitentiary. "We want to determine the numbers of inmates who are affected by prenatal alcohol, and see if the tool we use is effective as a screen for corrections officers," says Chudley. "The government wants to know the numbers so that they can appropriately plan programs in prison, and also do better planning for parole and aftercare." If the screening tool proves to be reliable, it might eventually also be used to identify (and thus help) high-risk individuals with FASD *before* they become involved in crime.

FASD, Race and Crime

In Canada, people of aboriginal background are far more likely to have FASD than those of non-native background, and six times as likely to be in prison. The Correctional Service Canada study says that although aboriginal people represent only 2 percent of the general Canadian population, they make up 13 percent of incarcerated offenders, and that similar statistics apply in the United States.

African-Americans make up about 13 percent of the U.S. population, but a whopping 60 percent of inmates in American prisons. In his meticulously researched book *Search and Destroy: African-American Males in the Criminal Justice System,* Jerome G. Miller points out that 75 percent of black American men, rightly or wrongly, acquire a criminal record by age the age of thirty-five. Miller examines many heart-breaking, racist reasons why African-American males are far more likely to be arrested, charged and convicted than are white males. However, he has overlooked one additional reason that many African-American men find themselves behind bars: according to a 1998 report by the Center for Disease Control in Atlanta, African-Americans are nearly seven times as likely to have fetal alcohol syndrome as are white Americans.

In New Zealand, the indigenous Maori represent only 14.5 percent of the population, but make up more than 50 percent of those imprisoned for non-traffic offences. Government statistics also indicate that 75 percent of all male inmates had suffered from alcohol abuse or dependence, and 84 percent had been drinking prior to a violent incident.[34] A recent survey indicates that although fewer Maori drink than in the general population, those that do so drink heavily. Forty-four percent of Maori male drinkers and 29 percent of Maori female drinkers consume alcohol at hazardous levels and are more likely to drink five or more drinks per occasion—enough to do substantial damage to the fetus.[35] As in the United States and Canada, inmates in New Zealand are almost never assessed for FASD.

Although Australia's native peoples are at high risk of both alcoholism and crime, corrections officials have never investigated the possibility of FASD among their Indigenous prison population. People of Aboriginal background and Torres Strait Islanders make up only 2.4 percent of the Australian population, but make up 19 percent of the prison population. In other words, their likelihood of being incarcer-

ated is about eight times as high as that of Australians of European heritage.[36] As in New Zealand, Indigenous Australians are more likely to
abstain from alcohol than other Australians, but those who do drink
are likely to drink at unsafe levels. Among Australians who do drink, 79
percent of Indigenous drinkers are heavy users of alcohol, compared to
12 percent of the drinkers in the general population.[37]

In recognizing the link between FAS and crime, the Canadian government is ahead of most countries in the world. New Zealand's
Christine Rogan of the government-funded Alcohol Healthwatch
wrote me a poignant note when she sent the statistics on Maori drinking and imprisonment:

> It paints a sad picture but we're currently unable to make any causal
> links with drinking during pregnancy. The Government is aware of
> FAS, and key Ministers were sent the Canadian Corrections report.
> We have been told that is it not significant enough to warrant any
> special consideration beyond general mental health therapy—let
> alone investigation and research.

FASD is not a problem restricted to any one race or class, but it's
certainly part of the cycle of poverty that affects aboriginal people all
over the world, and others whose cultures have been damaged or
destroyed. Poverty and despair are risk factors for alcohol consumption
in pregnancy, and emotional poverty and despair can affect anyone,
from the corporate wife to the pregnant street kid.

Presumed Guilty

Because they may behave oddly, and because they may be in the wrong
place at the wrong time, innocent people with FASD are often viewed
with suspicion by the police, and may find themselves arrested and
behind bars. Wanting to please the arresting officer, and unaware of
their rights, they may even confess to crimes they didn't commit.

Toronto's Margaret Sprenger fought a lengthy battle to help a long-time friend in his Kafkaesque battle with the law. "Russell," of native ancestry, removed from an alcoholic biological family, had been adopted into a family of professionals as a young child. Thirtyish, Russell looks much younger, and his excellent verbal skills, absorbed from his adoptive family, mask his severe learning disabilities. He had been homeless for many years, living out of a knapsack, poking through trash for "treasures," such as used electronic equipment.

One day in 1998 (three years before the September 11 tragedy) Russell was foraging outside a large shopping mall. Finding a large brown box full of government forms, all filled out, he realized that this material was confidential information. Trying to be a responsible citizen, he noted a Canadian flag flying outside the mall, and went inside to find the government office. Discovering a suburban courtroom, he took the box over to the security guard, plunked it down on the table, politely said, "I think you'll find this useful," turned and left.

Before reaching the exit, he was brought down by three security guards, who seized his knapsack, discovering a tangle of salvaged electronic parts, plus a plastic bag containing a mysterious white powder. This substance was sent to a lab, a bomb squad attacked the box, and Russell was interrogated at the police station. Nobody believed him. The white powder turned out to be instant mashed potatoes, often used by street people because it's a fast, filling, cheap source of carbohydrates. Russell was charged with public mischief. The case was remanded several times.

Margaret thought a diagnosis of FASD might be helpful, even though his legal aid lawyer was not interested in using it as a defence. Russell's adoptive parents could document his birth mother's alcoholism, and Russell has numerous physical and cognitive symptoms of FASD. But the doctor refused to give a diagnosis: Russell had once held a job for three months, and the doctor believed that a person with FASD is incapable of any kind of employment.

Because Russell had to have an address, he moved into Margaret's furnace room. Every week for fourteen months, he checked in with the bailiff. Every week, he visited a forensic psychiatrist, paid for by tax-payers. The psychiatrist diagnosed him with attention deficit problems and attempted to help Russell work on his "hidden anger." Russell told the psychiatrist, "But I'm not angry."

"Yes, you are," said the psychiatrist.

After being remanded several times, the case went to court on December 7, 1999—and the Crown withdrew charges. How much did this exercise cost the taxpayer for legal aid, the police officers' time, the bailiff, the forensic psychiatrist and the court costs? Russell told Margaret he had learned his lesson. He will never again try to be a good citizen. Next time he'll mind his own business.

Sexual Predators

We know that individuals with FASD are victims of sexual offences at a very high rate. Streissguth's secondary disabilities study says more than 70 percent have a history of being sexually abused at some point in their lives. So, if you have someone who has a history of early and inappropriate sexual behaviour, who is impulsive, who is easily led, it says to me that a number of them as adults would be involved in sexually related crimes.

—Jo Nanson

One case of sexual crime in which FASD was never mentioned was a 1999 trial that made international headlines. It combined Canada's national pastime of hockey with illicit sex and tragedy, in the historic Toronto sports shrine of Maple Leaf Gardens. Small, ugly, fifty-six-year-old John Paul Roby had worked as an usher in the Gardens for twenty-six years, and faced fifty-seven charges of sexually assaulting children, mostly boys, from the late 1960s to early 1990s.

Slight and uneducated, Roby had thick glasses, deep-set eyes, poor vision, a receding hairline and an odd-shaped face. One witness described him as being "a few bricks short of a load." He had many of the facial, physical and mental characteristics of fetal alcohol syndrome—three words that never came up at the trial. However, diagnosis might have been impossible, because there was no way of determining if Roby's mother drank in pregnancy: he had been abandoned at the door of a Quebec orphanage as a newborn infant.

The Crown prosecutor alleged that in return for hockey and basketball tickets, soda pop and ice cream, Roby had played sexual games, fondled the children, exposed himself and performed oral sex on countless occasions. The charges included gross indecency, indecent assault and sexual exploitation.

Questioned by his lawyer, the man who liked to describe himself as "Happy John" told of a childhood spent in various orphanages. Sexually assaulted by a Roman Catholic priest, he was later routinely beaten up and whipped at a work farm for orphaned children where he lived until age twenty. "We were told we were all mentally retarded and that's why we weren't in school."

A former altar boy, Roby had worked as a dishwasher, a salesman and a security guard before being hired in 1971, at twenty-eight, as an usher at Maple Leaf Gardens, where he worked around twelve hours a week in hockey season. For more than a quarter-century, he was a fixture in the "red seat" section, chatting with athletes and fans, collecting signed hockey sticks and other sports memorabilia—and allegedly using such souvenirs to lure boys to his home, where he would entice them to perform various sexual acts.

Roby pleaded not guilty to all fifty-seven charges. Convicted on thirty-five counts of sex crimes against minors, he was sent to Kingston Penitentiary and declared a dangerous offender who could never be released. On Thursday, November 8, 2001, the day before his lawyers were to file an appeal, he died suddenly of a heart attack at age fifty-eight, leaving the world as alone as he had entered it.[38]

Was the "monster of Maple Leaf Gardens" actually a lonely little man who was attracted to children because he, too, was mentally and emotionally a child? We'll never know if his horrific behaviour was the result of prenatal alcohol damage and a tragic childhood: despite numerous indications of FASD, the court never bothered to assess him.

The Worst Crime of All

The tragic eyes of Robbie Locklear look out from the mug shot of the North Carolina Department of Correction Public Access Information System website. His face resembles those of many of Colette's former street friends in the small, sad eyes, flattened midface and underdeveloped chin. The documentation is terse. "*Race:* Indian. *Birth date:* 05/16/1972. *Height:* 5' 6". *Weight:* 140. *Crime:* Murder first degree. *Total Term:* Death."

Robbie is Angelina Locklear-Taylor's beloved older son—and the man who murdered her husband, Jay. Angelina, one of seven children born to a Native American schoolteacher and his wife, was the family rebel. Her parents, members of the Lumby nation, were wealthy farm-owners in dirt-poor Robeson County, North Carolina. Although her parents and grandparents were teetotallers, Angelina tried her first beer at fourteen, moving quickly to bourbon and then to vodka, "'cause I thought nobody could smell it."

Although she drank frequently and rarely studied, Angelina was an excellent student. Despite her good grades, she didn't go to college, instead doing itinerant farm work. Robbie was born when she was twenty-one. His father was "just someone who had interested me when I was fourteen or fifteen . . . he never acknowledged Robbie."

Her baby was born one year before the *Lancet* study confirmed the link between maternal alcohol and birth defects. Despite Robbie's sweet disposition, he sometimes had an explosive temper, and had difficulty learning. When he started school his problems worsened. He began skipping classes, and the school would send him home as punishment.

In 1985, when Robbie was thirteen, Angelina became involved with "the love of her life," James "Jay" Charles Taylor. A white college teacher with two university degrees, he shared her love of knowledge—and alcohol, drinking tall Budweisers by the case. Their son,

J.R., miraculously not affected by alcohol, was born in 1987. By 1988 Angelina had sobered up, completed her college degree and become a social worker. Although Jay continued to drink heavily, she married him in 1991. By this time, Robbie, nineteen, with the mental age of a ten-year-old, had developed a drinking problem and had committed two petty crimes.

On the night of January 27, 1994, Angelina was working late, leaving Jay and her sons at home. While she was at work, little J.R., then seven, phoned to tell her that Robbie had shot his daddy—and within fifteen minutes, a police official called to tell her that Jay was dead.

Here's what Angelina has pieced together: proud of Angelina's six-year sobriety, Jay had been making an effort to quit drinking. Without alcohol, he had become increasingly miserable and difficult. Robbie was unemployed, broke and irritable. The two began to quarrel. Opening a king-size can of King Cobra beer, Jay threatened his stepson, "You better not be here when I get back," and went to the barn to get his rifle. He put his beer down to open the barn door—and Robbie shot him in the back with a shotgun someone had sold him for $10. Jay died instantly. Robbie was arrested and charged with murder.

A few months later, as lawyers prepared for the trial, Angelina, in her job as social worker, attended a presentation given by Susan Rich, a health professional who is now a medical doctor. "She talked to us about fetal alcohol syndrome—how people with FAS are slow to catch on, and mentioned some facial features and behaviour patterns. I was sitting there crying like a baby, thinking, 'she's talking about my son.'"

The trial jury consisted mostly of white men. It took them ninety minutes to issue a guilty verdict, convicting Robbie of first-degree murder; on May 14, 1996, two days before his twenty-fourth birthday, he was sentenced to death. "Race played a big part in the trial," says Angelina. "If my son and I had been white, and Jay had been Native American—instead of the other way around—this wouldn't have happened." As this book goes to press, Angelina's lawyers are requesting a new trial on the grounds of Robbie's mental disabilities and a diagnosis of FAS.

The Criminal Justice Industrial Complex

*It is characteristic of this form of punishment, inspired by all
that is pitiless, that is to say, brutalizing, that gradually, by a
process of mindless erosion, it turns a man into an animal,
sometimes a vicious one.*

—VICTOR HUGO, *LES MISÉRABLES*

More than 42 million people worldwide have seen the stage musical *Les
Miserables,* based on the epic novel about social justice by the nineteenth-
century French poet and novelist Victor Hugo. Watching the story of
Jean Valjean, imprisoned for nineteen years for stealing a loaf of bread,
audiences respond passionately to the tragedies portrayed on stage, but
do not connect these tragedies to the plight of people living in ignorance and poverty in the streets of their own cities, or incarcerated in
nearby jails, prisons and penitentiaries. In his book *Search and Destroy,*
Jerome Miller, who holds a doctorate in social work and has worked
extensively in juvenile justice, attacks what he calls the "criminal justice
industrial complex," which needs convicted bodies to fuel a multibillion-
dollar industry.

If Mr. Justice David Vickers of British Columbia had his way, we'd
be closing down jails instead. "If they build it, they will fill it," Vickers
told a packed workshop at the B.C. FAS conference in February 2001.
Justice Vickers takes every opportunity to develop alternative sentencing for non-violent offenders with FASD, addiction issues or other
mental health problems. He once forced a prosecutor and defence
lawyer to work together to have an offender assessed for FASD, then
ordered them to create a supportive community circle for the young
man for the next five years, so he could stay out of prison, thereby saving the taxpayers several hundred thousand dollars.

Vickers and many others point out that those 25 percent or more of
offenders who are living with FASD learn very little from being
incarcerated. Lacking insight, unable to learn from experience, they
learn instead to take violence for granted. On release they often find

213

themselves unemployable and homeless, and are likely to reoffend over and over.

American statistics indicate that crime victims in the United States lose about $18 billion per year as a direct cost of crime: losses of cash or property, medical expenses and lost pay resulting from injuries or activities related to the crime. Canadian statistics indicate that about one-third of robbery offenders were under the influence of alcohol or drugs on the day they committed the offence.

According to Canada's National Crime Prevention Strategy website, jailing offenders costs $50,000 to $80,000 per year per person (and $100,000 per year per Canadian young offender) and generally does little to turn an offender's life around. The United States incarcerates more people than any other industrialized democracy—600 inmates per 100,000 population (i.e., six out of every thousand Americans are in prison). Canada, with about 130 inmates per 100,000 population, comes second, spending about $10 billion annually for police services, the courts, legal aid and the warehousing of people in prisons and penitentiaries.[39] American taxpayers pay nearly $150 billion annually for criminal justice costs—half again as much per capita as Canadians—about $2,000 for every family of four.[40] Adding costs of security, insurance, loss, damage or being a victim brings the numbers close to $500 billion—about 7 percent of the U.S. gross national product.

In California, one of the states with the "three-strikes-you're-in-for-life" laws, 57 percent of inmates serving life sentences have been imprisoned for non-violent offences.[41] In an article in the *New York Times,* Greg Winter wrote of California "lifers" who have been permanently incarcerated for shoplifting items as small as Kmart notions, or four chocolate chip cookies.[42] Around Christmas 1999, twenty-nine-year-old Kenneth Payne stole a one-dollar Snickers bar from a Texas grocery store and was sentenced to sixteen years because he had been on probation for stealing Oreo cookies at the time; jailing him will cost the taxpayers a minimum of $800,000.[43]

My goal is that within ten years, Canada will be the first country in the world to close a jail. (The Honourable Claudette Bradshaw, federal secretary of state for homelessness, March 2003)

Mrs. Bradshaw, who spent more than twenty years working with children with FASD, understands the connections between alcohol and poverty, homelessness, abuse, addiction and crime. Like her, I believe that over the long term, Canada and other countries in the industrialized world could cut criminal justice budgets by at least 25 percent if we developed effective methods of supporting women in abstaining from alcohol in pregnancy. We'd see results even sooner if we

- developed diagnostic clinics and appropriate special education programs for all children and adolescents affected by FASD;
- routinely assessed every offender whose family history indicates a possibility of fetal alcohol damage; and
- created alternative methods of dealing with non-violent offenders with FASD.

Finally, we need to remember that most prisoners will eventually be released. Without an external brain, those with FASD—25 percent or more—are likely to commit more offences. They would be far better off, as would the general public, if they were offered knowledgable help for substance abuse, were taught a hands-on trade and, on release, were assisted in finding adequate housing and supportive employers. As the great Victor Hugo also wrote, "A man may leave prison, but he is still condemned."

CHAPTER TWELVE

The Puzzle of Pain Felt around the World

*She may have been raped. Especially being young girls, they try-
ing to heal their own problems. So they look for the first person to
come along . . . They drink beers an' wine, it is cheaper . . . They
get pregnant and then they forget to stop drinking. They have
money problems which leads to drinking, which leads to pregnancy, which leads to pension, which leads to drinking, which
leads to more problems which leads to more drinking, which leads
to more pregnancies—then they can't look after their kids.*

—AN AUSTRALIAN ABORIGINAL TEENAGER, QUOTED
BY THE EPIDEMIOLOGIST LORIAN HAYES IN HER
UNPUBLISHED PAPER, "GROG BABIES"

By 1999 Brian and I were corresponding with hundreds of parents
around the globe, including the United Kingdom, Australia, New
Zealand, Germany and South Africa. We knew that our children repre-
sented only the tip of Ann Streissguth's iceberg. Throughout the world,
official government statistics indicate deceptively low rates of births of
alcohol-affected children.

- In the U.S., the *Ninth Special Report to Congress on Alcohol and
  Health,* published by the National Institute on Alcohol Abuse

and Alcoholism, indicated that only 9.7 children per 10,000 are born with FAS—slightly less than one in 1,000.

- The 1998 Annual Report of the South Australian Birth Defects Register indicates that in this state (pop. 1.5 million) there have been *no* FAS births recorded since 1986. A foreword indicates that "prevalence rates of FAS in Australia are lower than in USA and Canada, and *this may reflect under-recognition, diagnostic difficulties and the fact that FAS is not reliably reported to birth registries*" (my italics).

- In spring 2000 New Zealand's minister of corrections decided to take no action on penal reform, based on a 1994 study that found only sixty-three children with FAS in the country's pediatric files.[44]

- Since the end of the second World War, alcohol consumption in Japan has shot up by 400 percent, yet this country claims a rate of FAS of only one in 10,000 births.[45] (Only severely damaged infants are diagnosed at birth.)

- No official Russian statistics seem available, but Jane Aronson, a New York doctor and adoption specialist, believes that at least fifteen Russian children in a thousand—1.5 percent—will have full FAS.[46] (This could mean that another forty-five to sixty per thousand will seem normal but will be affected by pFAS or ARND. In other words, at least 6 percent of Russian children are probably permanently affected by prenatal alcohol.)

- According to Irish cabinet minister Mary Coughlan, "The Irish are among the biggest boozers on the planet." She cites a recent study indicating that the annual cost of drug and alcohol-related harm is about 1.7 billion Irish pounds—more than 2 billion Canadian dollars.[47]

- In the United Kingdom, the Chief Medical Officer has indicated an increasing incidence of cirrhosis among women in their twenties— once only seen in women in their forties. The statement added that 27 percent of women and 15 percent of men are drinking more than the recommended weekly maximum of 14 units for women,

21 for men. The report also states that alcohol abuse costs British society an estimated £3 billion annually in absenteeism, unemployment, crime, accidents and premature deaths.[48] The costs of alcohol-affected children were not mentioned.

Rarely Diagnosed

The FAS specialist Donna Debolt explains that fetal alcohol damage is rarely diagnosed because "it's a disability that gets seen as children fail to meet their milestones." As infants and preschoolers, most alcohol-affected children fall within the normal range of development, she says. Their learning and behaviour problems only become obvious around age eight, and often reach crisis proportions by adolescence. But professionals tend to ignore possible birth defects when looking at teenagers, instead focusing on the youngsters' environments and current family dynamics. "Nobody ever goes back and asks what part of the adolescent's problems relate to prenatal exposure," says Debolt.[49]

She adds that only the most severely alcohol-affected infants will be diagnosed and reflected in official statistics, as pediatricians will spot them at birth. But the problems of seemingly healthy infants with FASD will not become evident until these children reach school age; they are seldom diagnosed or included in any statistics. Ann Streissguth and others estimate that about one in one hundred individuals in industrialized societies are affected by prenatal alcohol—about two in one thousand with full-blown FAS, the remainder with invisible pFAS or ARND.

International newspapers tell a story that is different from the official statistics. In our travels, or when reading foreign newspapers online, Brian and I constantly spot tragic stories about perpetrators or victims whose histories indicate undiagnosed fetal alcohol damage.

Our correspondence indicates a massive, unrecognized international problem. Only two of the children in this chapter are reflected in their country's official government statistics.

New Zealand

I am angry at the system. I battle constantly with authorities to attain recognition of FASD. This disbelief and lack of support in educating the public, and especially mothers-to-be, astounds me.
—SHIRLEY WINIKEREI, HAMILTON, NEW ZEALAND

When Shirley Winikerei of Hamilton, New Zealand, and her husband, Reuben, adopted five-week-old Demelza in 1977, Shirley was stunned by her first glimpse of the tiny girl. Shirley is *pakeha* (of European ancestry), her ex-husband of Maori descent. Baby Demelza, also of Maori background—from a large family the adoption worker described as "regular party-goers"—did not display the usual complexion or physical size or strength of the proud Maori race. Instead, she was "scrawny, lying stiffly in the bassinet . . . a sickly, pinky-fair color with fair hair." More than a quarter-century later, Shirley has become a feisty activist, known by Parliamentarians as "Shirley the Whinger" (pronounced "whinjer"—a down-under and British variant of "whiner").

Frequently hospitalized, baby Demelza suffered from breathing difficulties, constipation, allergies, skin rash and infections of urinary tract and ears. By ten months, she threw temper tantrums—screamed endlessly, rocked back and forth and hit her head on the wall (symptoms of "sensory integration" problems.) By three and a half she spoke only in unintelligible babble, requiring speech therapy. The doctors prescribed numerous medications for her—and antidepressants for Shirley, to help her cope with the stress of raising this difficult, sickly, child.

In primary school, Demelza, like Colette, displayed a great deal of independence and made friends easily, but her relationships did not last. She was disruptive in class—fidgeting, singing and moving around—but good at math, near the average in her other subjects and, despite her bad asthma, an excellent runner.

At nine, Demelza was banned from the local shopping mall for shoplifting. By ten, she was sexually promiscuous, refusing to use contraception. At eleven, she was fighting with boys and girls, and would sneak out of her bedroom at night. By this time the youth section of the local police and welfare agencies had become involved, and Shirley's marriage had collapsed.

Then Shirley saw a documentary about the author Michael Dorris and his book *The Broken Cord*. Sobbing as she recognized many of Demelza's behaviours, Shirley nevertheless went into denial. Because Demelza did not have the facial features commonly associated with FAS, "I just couldn't believe that alcohol could have done so much damage to her brain."

By high school Demelza was permanently truant, abusing alcohol and marijuana, sniffing glue and having dangerous rages. Shirley spent most nights searching for her daughter and her days coping with authorities who blamed her for her daughter's behaviour, wrongly attributing it to Demelza's having been sexually abused as a child. When Demelza destroyed her room and attempted to slash her wrists because she was not allowed to have a keg party, Shirley finally acknowledged that her daughter was affected by prenatal alcohol. In 1993 she met Ann Streissguth, who was doing a seminar at the medical school in Auckland. A friendship was launched that continues to this day.

At fourteen, Demelza became pregnant, binge-drinking throughout, and refused to terminate the pregnancy or give the child up for adoption. Her eight-pound baby girl, Kahurangi, was born in 1992, and Shirley has raised her since infancy. At first she seemed healthy, but then began to display all of the symptoms of fetal alcohol damage that had affected her mother, including tantrums, head-banging and sleeplessness. Demelza has given birth to four more damaged children by three different fathers, all in the care of child protection authorities. The men in Demelza's life tend to be alcoholic, abusive and in and out of jail for violent offences—probable victims of prenatal alcohol as well.

Over the past decade, Shirley has fought countless battles for alcohol-affected children and adults in New Zealand. Like Demelza, her granddaughter Kahurangi, now hitting adolescence, sometimes displays terrifying, explosive "murderous rages," which no medication can control. However, Shirley's knowledge of strategies for FASD has so far prevented the kind of delinquency seen in Kahurangi's mother. On a trip to New Zealand in 2003, Brian and I spent several days with Kahurangi and Shirley, and visited Shirley's famous office in her garage, which houses the Fetal Alcohol Support Trust, a non-profit organization that builds awareness and supports families. We were charmed by the young girl, and marvelled both at their close relationship and at Shirley's skills in dealing with her.

Australia

There is an urgent need in Australia for improved diagnosis of the disorder and for health professionals with specific training and experience in managing the core disabilities of FAS spectrum disorders. This group of people with disabilities should receive the same quality of care that is currently provided to those with other more visible and familiar disabilities.

—SUE MIERS, NATIONAL ORGANIZATION FOR
FETAL ALCOHOL SYNDROME AND RELATED DISORDERS
(NOFASARD), ADELAIDE, AUSTRALIA

While Brian and I struggled with adolescent Colette, Sue and Tony Miers of Adelaide, Australia, were caught in an almost identical family drama. Their daughter Lola and Colette were born within months of each other, and both were placed as infants with older foster parents until they found permanent homes. Sue was a former dental nurse/radiographer; her husband, Tony, a public servant. The couple had three older children, all preschoolers.

Of Aboriginal background, Lola was twenty months old when she became the Miers' long-term foster child. She seemed physically and mentally healthy. Like us, Sue and Tony were informed that their daughter's birth mother had been an alcoholic, but "I knew nothing about FAS or that alcohol affected the fetus," Sue says. "In fact, when I went through my pregnancies, nobody told me that either."

Toddler Lola couldn't learn nursery rhymes or colours, or under-stand *no*. She frequently burst into tears for no apparent reason. Now realizing that the tearful outbursts were the result of neurological over-load, Sue regrets listening to friends and family comment, "Oh, she's just drawing attention to herself."

Fearless, Lola would wander away from home if she wasn't con-stantly supervised, and would repeatedly clamber up a high trellis, despite warnings from her parents. In school, she was assessed with borderline intellectual disability but showed inconsistent competen-cies. Constantly in trouble, "she was a really beautiful, loving child, but she just didn't seem to be able to follow the rules." Because of Lola's small size and developmental delays, she was unable to develop friend-ships with her peers and generally played with much younger children.

Like Shirley Winikerei in New Zealand, Sue Miers learned about FAS in 1990, through the work of Michael Dorris. Sue was reading a maga-zine article about Dorris, when "It hit me in the face—that's my child." Dorris's adopted son Abel shared ten-year-old Lola's learning and behav-iour problems, and a family history that included maternal drinking.

Sue took Lola to the local genetics clinic, where—as happened to Colette—a doctor measured her head and said she was normal, and didn't have fetal alcohol syndrome. But he gave Sue a document indi-cating that her daughter had "a mild form of fetal alcohol syndrome." (Ann Streissguth's research indicates that there are *no* mild forms of fetal alcohol disorders—all permanently affect the central nervous system.)

Unhappy with this assessment, Sue sought more reading material and help. "I did the rounds—drug and alcohol agencies, parenting groups, disability services, and nobody had heard of fetal alcohol syn-drome." Lola's problems worsened: she became sexually active while still very young, and found herself in trouble with the law as a result of her impulsive behaviour. She left school in the eleventh grade, and tried several government-sponsored work placements, all of which broke down. Sue now realizes that in every job, Lola had been "set up for fail-ure because there wasn't enough supervision or structure."

In 1997, when Colette was panhandling on the streets of Toronto,

Lola was beginning to experiment with drugs, and Sue hit the Internet. Learning about Canada's first Prairie North conference on FAS in Calgary in 1999, featuring star speakers Dr. Ann Streissguth and Dr. Sterling Clarren, she decided to attend. Sue and I met in Calgary—Sue lugging a thick file on Lola, looking for a doctor who would diagnose Lola long distance. She found a Canadian diagnostician who was sympathetic, but he could not diagnose without seeing Lola. However, he looked over the file and told Sue that Lola's family history, learning and behavioural problems were consistent with at least partial fetal alcohol syndrome (pFAS).

Sue now knew that the "milder" end of the FAS spectrum is statistically more debilitating than the full syndrome. Returning to Australia, she founded the National Organisation for Fetal Alcohol Syndrome and Related Disorders (NOFASARD). Since then, she has worked to build awareness in a country whose history is linked with alcohol—a country where 160 wineries are owned by doctors who are proud to "imbibe what they prescribe."

Government agencies and academics in Australia have tended to ignore three decades of U.S. research, preferring to believe that FASD is virtually non-existent, despite the high national consumption of alcohol. The Australian anthropologist Maggie Brady has written numerous well-researched studies of Aboriginal communities, including two books on Aboriginal use of "grog." In her 1991 report, *The Health of Young Aborigines,* she makes frequent comparisons to young indigenous North Americans. At both ends of the earth, adolescents and young adults of native background are similar in their addictions to alcohol and gasoline-sniffing ("petrol-sniffing" in Australia) and their high fertility rates. Brady notes their frequent learning problems, high rates of school dropout, promiscuity, crime, suicide and accidental death. However, she has not recognized the links between alcohol use and the secondary disabilities of FASD; these disabilities are found on almost every page of her study—but not understood:

> Foetal Alcohol Syndrome (FAS), which is of grave concern in the U.S.
> and Canada among native people appears not to have had a major

impact as yet among Aboriginal people. For example, the Aboriginal medical service Pika Wiya in Port Augusta (rural South Australia) has noted only three cases of FAS out of 119 Aboriginal pregnancies on its books.[50]

"Only" three cases of FAS in 119 births is a shocking rate of nearly 3 percent, almost fifteen times the one-in-five-hundred rate that Streissguth and others consider to be the rate in many industrialized countries. U.S. researchers believe that for every case of full fetal alcohol syndrome in a community, there are at least three individuals living with subtle but devastating pFAS/ARND. Therefore, there is a high probability that at least another nine apparently normal children in this small community will probably never be diagnosed—for a total of twelve alcohol-affected children in 119 births, or 10 percent.

This rate is identical to the numbers found by Ab Chudley and Michael Moffatt in their 1997 study of an aboriginal reserve in Manitoba (see page 49). Assessing 179 children, Chudley and Moffatt identified eleven children with FAS and six with FAE, and wrote that for each of those seventeen children there were probably another two to three (a total of thirty-four to fifty-one) with behavioural and learning problems caused by prenatal exposure to alcohol. Dr. Moffatt was quoted as saying that "the world frequency of fetal alcohol syndrome in live births is one to three cases in 1,000. . . . We're talking roughly 100 cases of FAS/FAE per 1,000 births on the reserve, and that qualifies as an epidemic."[51]

Three full FAS births out of 119 in Pika Wiya indicates an epidemic as well. If those three children had flippers instead of arms—rather than invisible neurological damage—the authorities would be doing everything possible to inform the local citizens, prevent further birth defects and put in place resources for those children and their families. Yet children with defective limbs can often lead fairly normal lives; children with permanent brain damage cannot.

The epidemiologist Lorian Hayes, of Aboriginal background, is one of the few Australian professionals who are aware of the tragedy of

FASD. In her unpublished study, "Grog Babies," Ms. Hayes looked at the reasons young women drink alcohol during pregnancy. Interviewing twenty young women and twelve young men aged fourteen to twenty-five, all of Aboriginal background, some in a remote community, others in an urban centre, she found that *drinking behaviour begins at eight years old.* She also learned that most health professionals "had little knowledge of fetal alcohol syndrome or the effects of alcohol on the fetus." When she interviewed local midwives and nurses for her study, "they just looked at me with blank faces." Pediatricians "said that they can't do anything so why diagnose it—we'd only be stigmatizing mother and child."

Sue Miers's research convinced her of the huge incidence of undiagnosed FASD in Australia's Aboriginal communities, and in the non-Aboriginal community as well. As a result of Sue's work, a task force on fetal alcohol in the State of Southern Australia has been formed, looking only at prevention. No effort is currently being made to improve diagnosis or to develop programs for alcohol-affected children, adults or families. She's had little luck with the Australian media, who "don't even want to take it up. I've had approaches from all sorts of journalists who have worked on it, then nothing happens. Someone somewhere is influencing them, I'm sure."

Sue's knowledge enabled her to help Lola find work as a kitchen hand in a church conference centre, where her employers took the trouble to learn about FASD. They made allowances for "off days," sensory overload and memory problems, and gave her lists of things to do. But by the age of twenty-one, Lola had moved in with her equally disabled boyfriend. She was drinking heavily, prone to psychotic rages and cutting her arms (often a sign of borderline personality disorder.) She lost her job, was physically abused by her boyfriend and wound up in a hospital psychiatric ward, where staffers knew nothing about FASD.

Sue and Tony sought advice from the University of Washington Fetal Alcohol and Drug Unit. The researchers there believed that Lola needed to be in a residential environment for people with mental health problems, and would require this support indefinitely. An Australian psychiatrist agreed. Sue and Tony decided it was time for the government to step in. In a letter to the Intellectual Disabilities Services Council, they pointed out that as foster parents, they were no longer legally responsible for Lola as an adult.

Unfortunately, government officials referred Lola to professionals who failed to understand that she is often incapable of making informed decisions, and encouraged her to move to an independent living situation. Lola's heavy drinking increased. Eventually she was assaulted by two "friends" and, terrified, moved back to her parents' home.

In late 2003, Sue visited Brian and me en route to a conference on FASD in Winnipeg—this time paid for by the state of South Australia. Over tea in my kitchen, we recalled our first meeting in Calgary in 1999, and how she had returned to a country where most professionals denied that fetal alcohol was a problem. Partly due to her continuing efforts, she is now seeing increased interest in FASD. Several health agencies are beginning to study the incidence of prenatal alcohol damage; and a national reference group of interested professionals is emerging, with a goal of working for change. Although for several years she had little luck with interesting the media in the issue of FASD, a fine article had appeared in a national newspaper earlier that week, written by a bright young woman journalist.

Sue told me about the wonderful placement she had been able to secure for Lola in a large, supported living facility that provides full-time staff and recreation resources such as a swimming pool. Unfortunately, despite taking Naltrexone to control her addiction to alcohol, Lola was evicted because of alcohol use, volunteered to go to a rehab unit, checked herself out two weeks later—and the roller-coaster continues. Recognizing that she has done everything possible to help her daughter, Sue has decided to focus her energy on building awareness and helping other families. "Tony and I have to accept that we might not be able to break the cycle," Sue sighed. "We gave her twenty-three good years which she would not have had without us. There's nothing more we can do."

Japan

As a newborn, my niece Hiromi looked like any other new baby, and weighed just under eight pounds (3625 gm) at birth. . . . She would jerk her head and stretch backward with a cry . . . Hiromi's cries were a soft, "Ah, ah, ah," and the sound only lasted four or five seconds, with the rest of her crying in a silent mouthing. She also had a limp right eye. It would close and she would not be able to open it even if her left eye was wide open . . . these were all neurological signs that something was wrong.

—PEGGY SEO OBA, WEBSITE "FAS IN JAPAN"

Peggy Oba of Kansas City, Missouri, is third-generation Japanese-American. Her husband Ken, born and raised in Tokyo, has lived in the United States since 1979, and their daughter, Mari, was born in 1984. And in 1989 Ken's brother in Japan and his elegant wife, Masako, became proud parents of little Hiromi.

When Hiromi was born, Ken's father in Japan sent his American family many videos of his baby granddaughter. Peggy, watching those videos, was worried. The baby didn't seem quite normal. "She just nodded—she would suddenly fold over like a flower." Peggy, a dental hygienist, began using her medical skills to investigate what might be wrong.

She talked to a representative of her local cerebral palsy organization, who asked, "Did she smile at six weeks?"

"I said no, because in the early pictures she's very solemn, and then suddenly at three months she's smiling with one side of her mouth. They told me that if a child cannot smile at six to eight weeks there's probably some neurological damage." Watching the tapes repeatedly, Peggy noticed that the baby had "little staring things—absences. She would look off somewhere and suddenly disappear. We called it her disappearing act."

Peggy suggests that everyone dealing with children with FASD should make frequent videotapes, to pick up "behaviours or mannerisms that you catch out of the corner of your eye." The videos showed that her niece might suddenly kick, jerk her head several times, make a fuss and suddenly quiet down. Observers might think she was acting up—"But the videos show that her eyes roll up in the top of her head." Watching and re-watching, Peggy saw "both cerebral palsy and epilepsy occur together in the same child."

In February 1992 an article about FAS appeared in the *National Geographic,* accompanied by photos of children with FAS, and Peggy instantly recognized the face of FAS in Hiromi. As well, little Hiromi was late on all of her milestones—sitting up, teething, crawling, walking. She had an odd one-sided crawl, known as a "Bunny Hop," and when she began walking, she walked on her toes—both traits often seen in children with full-blown FAS.

Reading *The Broken Cord,* Peggy recognized her niece on every page. As Shirley Winikerei and Sue Miers had done, she wrote to the University of Washington's Fetal Alcohol and Drug Unit, whose information confirmed her belief. Reviewing the videos again, she noticed Masako's heavy drinking for the first time. On one occasion, she imbibed six drinks over dinner.

Shortly after Hiromi's third birthday, Masako was thrilled to announce she was pregnant with twins. Ken, visiting Japan at the time, warned Masako about drinking in pregnancy, but she giggled, "Americans doctors are so funny! They worry about everything!" and continued to drink heavily. Masako was hospitalized during the last trimester because the babies were not growing. In March 1994 Ken and Peggy received videotapes of the fraternal twins, a boy and girl. "The little boy had hair all over his face—another FAS symptom—and they hardly cried. Even at three days old, babies have a tendency to try to look for you. These kids were kind of blank-eyed." Despite numerous symptoms of FAS, the babies were not diagnosed.

Desolate at having been unable to protect her niece and nephew, Peggy went up to the University of Wisconsin and took three courses on FAS and addictions. "I learned that my sister-in-law has more societal and cultural problems than I would ever care to deal with," Peggy says. "She has dealt with them in the only way she knows how, and that is by drinking."

At one conference, Peggy was able to show photos of her nieces and nephew to Dr. Sterling Clarren. She explained that they were the children of relatives in Japan. "I don't diagnose kids unless I see them in person," Clarren told her, "but I strongly suggest that these children see a geneticist as soon as possible."

"So you're not going to tell me if it's FAS?" Peggy asked.

Clarren looked off in the distance, way beyond Peggy, and said, "I can't say anything, but I think you have a real gift for diagnosis."

Peggy's older niece, Hiromi, who is entering adolescence as I write this book, has had academic problems and has been sent to a private school. The twins have both had problems with toilet training, and her nephew is often violent, unable to function normally, his emaciated body in constant motion. When he was three, Peggy saw him viciously beating a chair that he had bumped into. "There was a look of such murderous rage on his face, seldom seen in a child or adult." At five he began grabbing women's breasts and other parts of their bodies. All efforts to stop this behaviour have failed. (Shirley Winikerei, describing her granddaughter; Lynn Frank, in chapter 9, speaking about her son, Adam; and Angelina Taylor, describing her son Robbie on death row, used the same term—sudden "murderous rages"—and like Peggy's nephew, Lynn's son, Adam, also exhibited a precocious interest in sex when he was nine.)

The children's grandparents make remarks that Peggy has seen countless times in FASlink letters—"one child is stubborn, another won't (or can't) listen, how smart the kids are at home but don't seem to cut it at school . . . What is amazing to our family is the similarities of the problems, even though the children come from all over the world. What is also the same is the unbelief, the difficulties in getting help and the unrelenting sorrow of the families."

In trying to create awareness of FAS in Japan, Peggy has been up against the same denial and lack of interest from the media as that experienced by Shirley in New Zealand and Sue in Australia. She has written to several newspaper reporters, and e-mailed newspaper websites, but in vain. She wrote to the (U.S.) National Institute of Alcohol Abuse and

Alcoholism, asking if they had any ties with Japan. Their only contact, a retired gentleman, sent her three studies showing that drinking among Japanese women is increasing rapidly—but he added that "due to concern and knowledge there were 'no unhappy babies in Japan.'"

Peggy has sent numerous letters and information packets to Japanese organizations and to a woman professor who had written a widely-read book on Japanese women. "She told me that drinking among women was a problem but refused to meet me in Tokyo to discuss the issue." Letters to several Japanese universities, the Japanese Ambassador to the United States and Japan's premier FAS researcher produced equally polite but noncommittal replies.

Peggy continues to research both FASD and women's role in Japan. Bright women like her sister-in-law, Masako, are discouraged from the kind of education that Peggy and her daughter, Mari, take for granted. "There's an old saying in Japan: 'Any woman with more than two years of college is over-educated.'" Peggy feels that many intelligent Japanese women, lacking options, encouragement and self-esteem, turn to alcohol for solace.

She has given presentations on FASD at conferences in Hong Kong, in Kuala Lumpur, Malaysia, in Singapore, and in Sydney, Australia. And like Sue Miers' efforts in Australia, her perseverance is beginning to pay off. As a result of Peggy's many letters, and the popularity of her Japanese-language website, the ASK (Human Care) foundation, sponsored by the Japanese brewers association, held the first Japanese/Asian FAS conference in Tokyo on November 8th, 2003. Peggy helped them find the main speakers, both high-profile American specialists in FASD. "I was invited to do a presentation on 'my office,'" she chuckles. "As it's a corner of my daughter's bedroom, filled with cardboard boxes and stacks of paper, I declined."

Germany

I've lived in Germany for twenty years, and I'm still astounded by the amount of alcohol that gets drunk here. You cannot go anywhere—even school or church—without having beer available. When people come to my house to pick up their children at birthday parties, I offer them a tea or a coffee or a water—anywhere else they go the parents have got a couple of crates of beer. It's beer, it's classed as a food!

—ANN GIBSON, KIEL, GERMANY

Ann Gibson, a foster parent in Kiel, Germany, received a call from her social worker one Thursday afternoon in 1989. "We've got a four-month-old baby with *fasalkoholembryopathie* (FAS) in the Kinder clinic," the worker told her, "and if you don't take her she'll have to go into a home on Monday."

Ann knew nothing about FAS. "We thought children with alcohol damage were a little bit behind and would catch up." But she realized that when the worker talked of putting this baby in a "home," she meant an *orphanage*, and she could not let that happen. The following week the fragile, blond, blue-eyed Sinja (pronounced "Sinya") became a "temporary" member of the British expatriate Gibson family—joining Ann, husband, Alan, their three daughters (then aged seventeen, fifteen and twelve) and foster son, Andy, seven, who has a rare genetic disease called Rubinstein Taybi Syndrome.

Ann was told that Sinja would be there for only six months, until her twenty-seven-year-old mother had finished treatment for her alcoholism. However, the mother relapsed almost immediately, and the Gibsons were asked to keep Sinja permanently, as foster care in Germany is generally a permanent arrangement. (Sinja's birth mother died in 1997 of cirrhosis.)

At four months old, Sinja was the size of a newborn, and would arch her back and scream for hours on end—a behaviour that doctors attributed to withdrawal from alcohol. Because Sinja had a cleft palate,

231

and had difficulty in sucking from a bottle, she had to be fed through a nasal gastric tube, which she kept pulling out. She couldn't stand to be cuddled, and feeding her was a nightmare. The entire family were sleepless wrecks. Finally, at eight months, she began to use the bottle. Prepared baby foods were another challenge. Because of her cleft palate, the food often came out her nose. Three operations were required to close the palate—at one, three, and five years old.

Shortly before her seventh birthday, Sinja was tested by a psychologist, who told the Gibsons that she needed to go to a school for the mentally disabled. Ann knew that their daughter was too bright for that kind of school. "For the first time, we realized that FAS wasn't going to go away. We'd hoped that if we worked enough with her, she'd become normal."

Fortunately, Kiel is near the German–Danish border, and Ann's other children had attended Danish-language schools. A nearby Danish public school had three classrooms for learning-disabled children, and Sinja was enrolled at age eight. Now an adolescent, Sinja is fluently trilingual—in English, Danish and German. For parents of FASD children who have battled North American school systems, Sinja's Danish language school sounds like a bit of heaven. The school is small (three hundred pupils), with a family atmosphere, in which "teachers, pupils and parents are on first-name terms."

There are about six to ten children in the special education classes. "They have a structured timetable, but occasionally make room for spontaneous activities such as nature walks, or even trips to the ice cream café if they've been especially good!" Sinja will continue with this school until she completes tenth grade. Teachers have been willing to learn about the problems of each child. "They still get frustrated that she can recognize a letter or number one day and forget it the next. But they work just as we do at home—repeat, repeat, repeat!"

When Sinja was nine, X-rays of her left hand indicated that she had the bone age of a four-year-old. The Gibsons were told that without hormones, she would never be taller than 143 centimetres—about four foot eight. Because so many fat cells were destroyed in utero, she eats like a trucker without gaining weight, and because she is so thin, she always feels cold. Sinja continued taking growth hormones until she reached five foot two (159 cm) in early 2003, aged fourteen.

Having two disabled foster children in Germany entitles the Gibsons to respite unavailable in North America. For four weeks every year, the German government pays a trained caregiver to look after their children—while stressed-out parents go to a special hotel with a swimming pool and excellent food, at a cost of about $100 U.S. per couple. Most government officials in North America believe that we can't afford the resources for families of disabled children that the Gibsons receive in Germany. It's possible the postwar German economy has been so successful because all children—even those as fragile as Sinja—have been viewed as important human beings and treated accordingly.

Like Shirley Winikerei and Sue Miers, Ann Gibson has become a national advocate on issues relating to FASD. Working in her second language, she founded FASworld Deutschland, using her creativity to build a country-wide organization providing support and information. She has also helped to develop FASeurope, an international body that currently has members from Germany, England, Ireland, Scotland, Luxembourg, Poland, Sweden, the Netherlands and Austria.

South Africa

The incidence [of FAS] is higher in poor communities and in socially marginalised groups featuring high rates of alcoholism. These conditions are typical in many parts of the Western Cape, and are compounded by a culture of heavy drinking, especially in wine growing areas, Prof. Viljoen [of the University of Cape Town and South Africa's leading authority on FASD] said. "These factors are producing what may be the highest fetal alcohol syndrome rate in the world." . . . He has found . . . that about 20 percent of children in a particular pre-school in Philippi have full-blown fetal alcohol syndrome.

For every child with full-blown fetal alcohol syndrome, there are probably five with fetal alcohol effects . . . Professor Viljoen believes that between 5 000 and 10 000 children are born every year in the Western Cape with some form of fetal alcohol syndrome, almost all of them in the poorest communities.
—UNIVERSITY OF CAPE TOWN NEWSLETTER, MARCH 3, 1997

One of my favourite photos is of blond, beaming Vivien Lourens of Cape Town, nose to nose with her impish, ebony-skinned little daughter, Tisha, who was three years old when the picture was taken. Vivien, a British expatriate, immigrated to South Africa in 1974, and met and married the Dutch-born Peter Lourens, a mill supervisor who had immigrated in 1965. Like the Gibsons, Vivien and Peter are foster parents whose hearts always have room for another child. Of Cape Coloured background (a mixture of white European and black African heritage), Tisha arrived in the Lourens household at the age of ten weeks as a "temporary" emergency foster placement, straight out of hospital. When Vivien took Tisha for her four-month checkup six weeks later, she was told, "Oh, she's FAS, you know."

Like Sue in Australia, Vivien began looking up FAS information on the Internet. At first, doctors told her, "This child probably won't live." But Tisha did live, and Vivien was then told that the little girl wouldn't walk until she was five. Defying predictions, Tisha took her first steps at one year and was walking by eighteen months.

Tisha's mother, who vanished long ago, was alcoholic, asthmatic and tubercular; she lived in one of the worst "camps" in the Cape Town area. Vivien suspects she may be dead, and believes that she may also have had FASD. "Tisha probably wouldn't have lived if she had stayed with her biological mother," Vivien reflects.

By the time Tisha was a year old, the family had put a lot of work and love into helping her prove the doctors wrong, and there "was still nobody for her. Nobody would take a 'special needs child,' so she would have to go into a children's home." Like Ann and Alan Gibson in Germany, Vivien and Peter could not let this happen—and Tisha stayed.

Vivien and Peter have an adolescent son, David, and Vivien also has

234

an older son and three grandchildren by a previous marriage, all living in the United States. They have two other school-age daughters—one foster, one adopted—and temporary foster infants come and go. In this chaotic household, Tisha, with her sparkling personality and "wonderful, dry sense of humour" lights up everyone's life.

As an emergency foster mother, Vivien looks after the infants until health or other problems have been sorted out, and then the children go into permanent foster care, or are adopted. Tisha, now school age, is a permanent foster child. As in other countries, adopting would mean losing funding for her medicine and other expenses. "It's purely a financial thing because, boy, if they tried to take my child away from me, I'd kill them!"

All the children go by the surname Lourens. The income from foster care isn't much, but in cash-strapped South Africa it's very useful. Vivien gets nine rands (about $1.62 Canadian) per day for each emergency foster child. The Lourens depend on the community to assist with second-hand baby clothing and items such as prams.

In South Africa, the huge disaster of FAS has taken a back seat to the pandemic of AIDS, which has resulted in 50,000 orphaned babies annually, many with AIDS themselves. Vivien Lourens cites statistics indicating that about 10,000 to 12,000 infants in South Africa are born with FAS annually, most of them the tragic result of the *dop* system, which is now illegal. For countless years, wineries paid their workers—generally Cape Coloured—partly in wine to compensate for very low salaries. Although this system has been discontinued, it left behind thousands, possibly hundreds of thousands, of alcoholics—many of whose addictions go back generations.

But those 12,000 new cases of FAS each year are only the tip of the iceberg. Another 30,000 to 40,000 children will be born with the invisible disabilities of pFAS/ARND, and will probably never be diagnosed. Because the 50,000 babies with AIDS are far more ill and visible, there are few resources for foster mothers of infants with FASD. "The formula for our babies has been taken away from me because the AIDS babies must have it."

Between 1998 and 2000, twenty-seven babies moved in and out of the Lourens household, nearly all of pure African or Cape Coloured background, and Vivien believes that many of these probably had FASD as well.

Frustrated by the lack of awareness of the tragedies resulting from prenatal alcohol, Vivien sighs at the endless, depressing cycle of poverty and alcoholism she sees around her every day. "When people say, 'How can they do this?'—well, you should see the conditions that some of these people live in. There are people a few miles away who are living in cardboard boxes," she says. "They don't have sanitation or electricity. They use gas lamps and fires, and if they accidentally set their shack on fire, by tomorrow we'll hear of another area that's burned to the ground. If I lived that way, I think I would drink as well."

The terrible living conditions Vivien describes, which contribute to alcoholism and fetal alcohol damage, are not unique to South Africa. This soul-crushing misery is found worldwide in aboriginal communities from Alaska and Arctic Canada, across North, Central and South America, to Australia and the Maori in New Zealand. Blotting out their pain, abused pregnant women are also drinking right now in tenements in the United Kingdom, shantytowns in the Caribbean, slums in Chicago, inner-city alleys behind the glittering high-rise towers of my home city of Toronto and decaying cities and towns throughout the countries of the former Soviet Union. In many of these areas, the almost invisible disability of FASD may seem dwarfed by the visible horror of AIDS/HIV.

But there's another kind of poverty: the emotional poverty encountered by Peggy Oba in her Japanese relatives. This kind shows up in affluent societies that have lost their way. Traditional institutions have crumbled and been replaced by a global economy that believes only in the human value measured in possessions. In middle- and upper-middle-class societies across the industrialized world, women who "need" to drink daily are known as moderate drinkers unless they are falling-down drunk. Their acting-out children are mysteriously afflicted with learning disabilities, dyslexia, attention-deficit hyperactivity disorder (ADHD) or conduct disorder. "People who drink have empty hearts and they use alcohol, drugs, material things and activities to fill them up, and the more they use, the emptier they get," Peggy wrote to me.

Back in the sixties, when fresh-faced idealists dared to hope, we had a saying: "If you aren't part of the solution, you're part of the problem."

Sue Miers, Shirley Winikerei, Peggy Oba, Ann Gibson and Vivien Lourens are part of the solution.

CHAPTER THIRTEEN

Marvels, Miracles and Dancing at the Mall

He is my son. He can drum, dance, sing. He has wonderful con-nections with the Higher Power somewhere, which is beyond my abilities to understand. My son will lay his hand on my cheek and say, "Mom, I love you so much." Brandan is an unbeliev-able miracle . . . all my children are.

—Julie Gelo, adoptive mother/caregiver
of seven children with FASD

When my kid begins to bug me at the mall I just start dancing. AND I'm forty-two years old and 220 pounds (imagine that). The whole thing just stops her cold and she knocks it off . . . there is great power in not caring any more what people think!

—Bunny, mother of Lindsay, age twelve

Certain parents have eyes that dance when they talk about their alcohol-affected children. One of these is social worker Kim Meawasige, whose tiny school-aged daughter Brenda has severe developmental delays, and doesn't understand the concept of time. "Whenever I'm away from her—whether it's been two days, or ten minutes in the laundry room—when I come back into the room, she's so glad to see me, she throws her-self at me and hugs me. She lights up my life!"

Now in their early thirties, Kim and her husband, Greg Flynn, are parents to six children—four adopted children with FAS, and two biological daughters, one of whom has severe juvenile arthritis. Kim, of Ojibwa heritage, takes great pride in the achievements of all of her children. One daughter is a talented "shawl dancer"; two other daughters, teenagers with FASD, have done well in high school, with extra support; her physically disabled daughter is a determined little fighter; her only son is a gifted artist; and impish Brenda never fails to make her laugh.

There are many other children with FASD who are beating the odds, and FASlink members were delighted when the ten-year-old biological son of moderator Bruce Ritchie in Sarnia won all five events in the local Boy Scout Kub Kar race. When Judy Pakozdy's son Matt, of the Yukon, graduated in dance from an elite college for performing arts. When Jodee Kulp's daughter Liz was named Adopted Child of the Year by the Minnesota Foster Care Association, and also received her Girl Scout Silver Award for her FASD efforts. And we rooted for tall, shy, twenty-three-year-old Tom Wilkinson when he and his black Labrador, Shadow, walked 1,800 kilometres (1,150 miles) through twenty-eight cities in southern Ontario, attempting to raise $1 million for an education and treatment centre for young people with FASD. (He raised $21,000—and a lot of awareness.) And when one of our children graduates from high school, college or university, the rest of us dare to hope, just a little.

Since early 1997, when I began communicating daily with hundreds of FASD families around the world, I've collected numerous success stories. Many of these parents were originally told that their children might never walk . . . or talk . . . or learn. Parents often use the word "miracle" to describe these tough little survivors. I think back to my failed search in my massive two-volume *Oxford English Dictionary* for the word "teratogen"—an agent that causes birth defects. The closest I could find was "teratogenesis"—the creation of monsters or marvels.

Some children with FASD may seem to be monsters, especially when parents, teachers and medical and social services professionals fail to recognize the extent of their neurological damage. Their learning disabilities can include difficulties both in school and in learning from experience. They may also exhibit poor judgment, an inability to respect other people's property, lack of impulse control, extreme mood swings, and seeming dishonesty. Some are so damaged that their behaviour puts their family at risk. In these instances, a well-supervised group home may be the only answer.

At the other end of the spectrum are "marvel" children whose parents view them as heroes—as Kim does. They may never learn to do algebra, but they are wonderful poets, artists, dancers, musicians, athletes or horseback riders. Some become Eagle Scouts or win Special Olympics medals or are, simply, fine human beings. The rest of us look on in envy, and frequently ask these Superparents for advice and support.

Teresa Kellerman and John

I've been parenting this boy-man for 24 years now and probably will for a few more years, until he is ready to enter a residential placement—or perhaps when I am ready for him to enter a residential placement. But I've been so successful in helping John become a respectable and socially acceptable adult that I actually enjoy his company. I never, ever thought I would make a statement like that, but I mean it—he is one wonderful guy!
—TERESA KELLERMAN, FAS FAMILY
RESOURCE CENTER, TUCSON, ARIZONA

When I first signed up with FASlink, I was captivated by the encyclopedic knowledge, creativity and quick wit of Teresa Kellerman of Tucson, Arizona. Creator of the world's most comprehensive website relating to fetal alcohol—the clever, constantly updated www.fasstar.com—-Teresa has also built websites for many other FASD activists. She is the single mother of two mentally disabled young adults: John, diagnosed with FAS as an infant, and fragile blond Karie, born in 1974, who has Prader-Willi syndrome (PWS). Because Karie's rare genetic disorder causes extreme developmental delays, psychiatric disorders, short stature, metabolic problems causing overweight and insatiable appetite, she needs constant monitoring, and has been in a group home since she was fifteen. John (a.k.a. Johnny) still lives at home, and Teresa's biological son, Chris, two years younger, recently graduated from university.

"When I first saw John, he looked not quite human, or not quite finished," Teresa says. Born one month prematurely, weighing less than three pounds, baby Johnny weighed only four pounds when Teresa, his emergency foster mother, took him home from the hospital in the fall of 1977. Johnny was eight weeks old and too small for "preemie" baby clothing, so Teresa dressed him in doll clothes and diapers that were cut in half. He had been diagnosed at birth with fetal alcohol syndrome, but Teresa could find nothing in the medical books about prognosis or intervention. Believing that "love is all you need," Teresa "took pride in taking special needs 'failure to thrive' babies and helping them to grow and thrive. All he needs, I thought, is my loving attention and my wonderful nurturing. Wrong!"

Baby John cried constantly, refused to be cuddled, rocked or sung to, and would only drink from his bottle if Teresa propped it, and left him alone in his crib in a quiet, dimly lit room. "During the early years, I struggled with getting him to eat, to gain weight, to sleep, to relax, to grow, to develop, to learn." Today, happy-go-lucky John devours his favourite snacks, would sleep until noon if she let him, and "shows no traces of the scrawny, screaming infant I was determined to save with my love." As a result of early diagnosis and Teresa's knowledge and determination, John has escaped nearly all of the secondary disabilities outlined in the Streissguth study.

> My definition of success for my son Chris, who is not alcohol-affected, is to finish college, get a decent job and raise a healthy, happy family without going into debt. My definition of success for John is to avoid imprisonment, addiction, homelessness, parenthood and accidental death.

Attending a workshop on secondary disabilities when John was eighteen, Teresa realized "I had done something right all these years." She put her "seven secrets to success" on the Internet, and now presents workshops across the United States, teaching her SCREAMS model of intervention strategies for children and adolescents with FASD: "Structure, Cues (John calls it 'nagging'), Role Models, Environment, Attitude, Medications and Supervision."

"The good news is these really work," says Teresa, "The bad news is they have to be in place every day for the rest of his life." John's IQ has been assessed at about 70. But with special help, particularly from his mom, he graduated from high school, has held several part-time jobs and is a talented drummer and a warm, delightful human being.

Meeting Teresa and John on a trip to Arizona in 1998, Brian and I were touched by his eagerness to learn more about us, and about Canada. He's charming, inquisitive and ethical, and we frequently glimpsed the person he would have become if not for prenatal alcohol: a philosopher, musician or a lawyer championing the rights of the oppressed.

We were saddened by his apparent loneliness, a problem for almost every young person with FASD. As a result, Teresa's many e-mail friends have been happily following the long-distance romance between John and a beautiful young woman with FAS in another state. After many visits back and forth and frequent e-mails and phone calls, they became engaged at Christmas 2002. With Teresa's encouragement, John has recognized that he would have great difficulty being a father, and has had a vasectomy. But with the guidance and support of their families, some of their other dreams may come true.

Chris Margetson and Joe

There's a wide spectrum of damage, and I know that Joe may not be as damaged as some kids—but he's more damaged than other kids. If Joe does the best he can with what he has, then

*other kids can do their best too. It's really important that we
continue to give families hope.*

—CHRIS MARGETSON

When eight-year-old Joe was diagnosed with FAS in 1988, Chris
Margetson became determined to do everything possible to ensure a
good life for her son, who had been affected by her drinking in pregnancy. She found few community resources, but through trial and error
was able to develop strategies that built on Joe's strengths. Now in his
early twenties, Joe works full time. His height, good looks and easy
charm mask the extent of his invisible disabilities. Through his
mother's efforts, Joe—like John Kellerman—has avoided the secondary
disabilities described in Ann Streissguth's study.

Chris's first step was to find a good school for Joe. His sister,
Amanda, five years older, is not alcohol-affected but was also experiencing problems in the Roman Catholic school system. When Chris
attempted to inform the principal and Joe's teacher about his disabilities, she was told, "There is no way in this school that we will ever be able
to meet Joe's needs." Deciding to remove both Joe and Amanda from
that system, Chris—a single mother—set to work finding alternatives.

Fifteen years after fetal alcohol syndrome had been defined, Chris
was still unable to find a definitive education program. Instead, she
cobbled together pieces of research that indicated that youngsters with
FAS did best with smaller class sizes and one-on-one teaching, that
computers were useful and that physical education was extremely
important. "Kids need a pattern of active and quiet time—a time to run
off their energy, and other time to be still." By looking at research
around other learning disabilities, and studying Joe, Chris began to
sense what he needed, but "realized pretty quickly that there was no
way in the public system that he was going to do well."

Chris visited several private schools and eventually found the King
Academy in Kitchener, a one-hour drive from her home. Located in a
large old house, the school was run by an experienced teacher with
a Ph.D. in psychology. After giving Joe a new psychoeducational

assessment, the school designed a program that matched his needs and abilities. Tuition fees were $8,000 per year, a lot of money in 1988, but Chris says, "If I had damaged this child, the least I could do was do everything in my power to give him the best chance for success."

Joe had the same teacher for the next four years, and there were only eight children in his class. Unusual for 1988, every child had a computer. There was no gym, but two half-days per week were designated for physical education using local gyms, swimming pools, tennis courts, skating rinks and ski hills. By Friday afternoon many youngsters were incapable of concentrating, so the principal dismissed them early to do something that interested them—arts and crafts, for example, or a sport. These "off-times" helped the children develop their interests and learn how to access community resources. Watching Joe blossom in this nurturing atmosphere, Chris learned how all of us should deal with children with FASD:

> We can't get the most from them without being emotionally linked to them. As long as they see us as the enemy, they're not going to be able to respond. As long as they see us as the ally, they'll do their best for us. . . . Joe perceived the adults in that school differently than he had ever perceived adults in his life before.

After four years, Chris could no longer afford to send Joe to private school, and the lengthy drive was wearing her out. However, she found an adequate eighth-grade class in the public system, and an excellent pilot project, a self-contained classroom for grades nine and ten in the regular high school. Here, Joe would have the same teacher for all of his academic subjects, but attend "mainstream" classes for optional subjects such as physical education, shop and music. Unfortunately, the pilot program was dismantled, and Joe did not complete his high school diploma.

Instead of nagging Joe about dropping out, Chris helped him to find a job in a nearby daycare centre, where the staff and children alike appreciated his energy and sunny nature. Chris used similar creativity to cope with other problems often inherent in alcohol-affected young-sters. She prevented Joe from "borrowing" from her by protecting him from opportunities to do so: even at home she kept her money and valuables in a fanny pack around her waist. When Joe began to smoke marijuana frequently, she found a therapist who counselled him on "harm reduction" for several years. Joe now works in recycling for a brewery, and has a driver's licence.

Using her own experience to help others, Chris has formed a small charitable organization called Fetal Alcohol Syndrome Assistance and Training (FASAT), which offers training programs to organizations across Canada. The only self-identified birth mother on the Canadian government's National Advisory Council on Fetal Alcohol Syndrome, she is always willing to talk with mothers who drank in pregnancy, and are desperate for nurturing support and advice.

The Barkers and Anne Marie

Anne Marie was shocked this week when her friend told her that, in school, when you take a test, you can't just say that you don't know the answer and have the teacher explain it to you. You have to guess and hope you're right. Being home-schooled, this sounded absurd to Anne Marie. She asked, dumbfounded, "Do they want you to feel bad because you don't know?"

—CLAUDIA BARKER

Since 1997 I have enjoyed Claudia Barker's e-mails about life on her family's three-acre mini-farm in tiny Bastrop, Texas, outside Austin. They have a fluffy white rooster named Bing Crosby, a pygmy goat and two giant coon hounds named Bubba and Daisy. Claudia's rusty white van bears the magnetic sign Ma Barker's Extra Fancy Children, Chickens, Eggs and Goats. Brian and I were delighted to meet her, her husband, Kelly, and their daughter, Anne Marie, on a trip to San Antonio in 2001.

Several years earlier, Claudia had sent me a photo of five-year-old Anne Marie, whose shiny dark Dutch-boy bob and sparkling brown eyes reminded me of my younger sister, when we were kids. But like many young females with FASD, Anne Marie, now nine, was approaching puberty early, and her sleek hair had become a mop of curls. Petite, shy and quiet, she padded along beside her parents as we explored San Antonio's famous River Walk, looking forward to dinner at Anne Marie's favourite Mexican restaurant.

The restaurant was brightly decorated and noisy, the food was wonderful, and the conversation bounced back and forth until Kelly said quietly, in mid-meal, "Anne Marie and I are going for a little walk."

As they slipped away from the table, Brian and I looked at Claudia quizzically. "The noise, the atmosphere—it was just a little too much for her," Claudia explained calmly, scooping more guacamole. "She was about to hit meltdown."

Claudia says that she and Kelly can now read the subtle signals that Anne Marie is becoming overstimulated. "She makes some kind of repetitive movement—kicking a table leg, tapping her fingers, hitting the heel of her hand on her head. You can almost hear a buzz from her; she's not focused but seems to be somewhere else." When a real meltdown begins, Anne Marie overreacts to something minor, then begins talking loudly, withdraws from people and might hit anyone who comes near or tries to touch her. She'll try to escape "under or inside something"; she drools and makes loud animal-like screams; she throws things and repetitively pounds on any surface or object. When it's over, she cries. Meek and exhausted, unable to remember exactly what she has just been doing, she then does her best clean to up the damage, "and is depressed and self-blaming."

Numerous FASlink posts deal with rages and tantrums that explode out of nowhere for seemingly no reason, and vanish as quickly as summer hailstones. Some psychologists, such as Carol Stark Kranowitz in her book *The Out-of-Sync Child*, attribute these outbursts to "sensory integration" problems—some odd circuitry in the individual's sensory processing machine. Children with sensory integration problems can be acutely sensitive or insensitive to various stimuli, and even have a combination of these extremes.

Three strategies have helped Claudia and Kelly to dramatically reduce the incidence of these events, which in many respects resemble epileptic seizures. First, Anne Marie was for many years on anti-convulsant medication (which she now cannot take as it seems to cause over-production of insulin). Second, her parents removed her from a school that was compounding the problem (teachers and principal failed to understand her disabilities). Finally, her parents and brothers can quickly recognize the signs of impending meltdown—and quickly change the environment to head it off.

Because the only local public school was unwilling to accommodate Anne Marie's special needs, Claudia was forced to home-school her daughter, and has done so since second grade. Holding a degree in speech and language from University of North Texas, Claudia also has a teaching certificate for kindergarten to twelfth grade, but says that all of this education was useless as she'd had no training in the learning disabilities of FASD. Before beginning to home-school, she examined all of Anne Marie's tests, to figure out how she learned best, and then bought several curriculum guides, which she later threw out.

"Teaching her was amazingly easy, compared with all the trouble that we went through with the school system—all the bad notes they sent home . . . and if a child got five red marks she'd be punished in some way." When they first began, Anne Marie was anxious and fearful of getting punished: "What if I don't finish this? Then what?" Claudia then developed strategies to help her learn without anxiety. She never tests Anne Marie, and when teaching something new, she begins with material "she knows real well" and builds on that knowledge, repeating material over and over. Anne Marie is good with computers, as they are visual. Claudia keeps a teacher's plan book, and documents both what she planned, and what was actually accomplished.

Because Anne Marie has hearing difficulties, and takes in much of her information by lip-reading, she had been disruptive in school when videos were shown. But Claudia quickly discovered that open-caption school videos, with all of the words printed on the screen, are a wonderful teaching tool. Funded by the U.S. government, the videos are available for every Disney movie and also on virtually every topic—history, geography, science, literature. Claudia recommends open-caption videos for any child who is having difficulty in learning to read.

The school had taught phonics, but as Anne Marie cannot hear the difference between many sounds, Claudia taught her to recognize words by sight. Anne Marie has become a good reader, "and unlike a lot of kids with fetal alcohol damage, her comprehension is good." Like many alcohol-affected children, Anne Marie has great difficulty remembering math facts—but she does understand the concepts of addition, subtraction, multiplication and division, so Claudia has taught her to work with a calculator.

Anne Marie loves science, and Claudia has field guides to everything. "She loves finding and identifying butterflies, birds, insects, grass, trees and flowers." To teach history and geography, Claudia used a series of books called American Girls, which looks at American history through the eyes of little girls in various historic periods—what they ate, how they lived. "We did that up to the Civil War, finishing with a little girl named Abby, who was a slave, and was emancipated."

Flexibility is the key: if Anne Marie becomes excited about a project, they'll stick with it all day. "Home-schooling becomes a way of life and not something that you start doing at eight o'clock and finish at three." Like many other people with FASD, Anne Marie has some unusual gifts. Her sense of smell compensates for her hearing problems: "She can walk into the barn and smell if a snake has been in there." And like Colette, she's exceptionally talented with animals.

Since Anne Marie was six, she and her mother have looked after their thirty-odd chickens. Their goal: to have one of every breed of chicken they could find. Claudia has taught Anne Marie how to graph egg production, and her daughter has also written about them, kept a book on their statistics, read chicken care books and gone online to learn more.

She can tell you all the details of every chicken: their names (Mary, Sarah, Stripey, Linda, Moe, Tuesday, etc.), their breed and its characteristics, where in the world that breed originated and the health history of that particular chicken. She knows how to spot chicken ailments (like bumble-foot, worms and fowl-pox) and usually knows when a chicken is ailing before I do. She can look at an egg and tell you which chicken laid it, and which nest it probably came from (they have their favorite nests). She talks to them.

Claudia draws a warm word-picture of the little girl who the teachers said could never learn. "She often sits at her little school desk with a chicken on her lap as she does her work, and they gently cluck back and forth to each other while she works. I doubt if I could get that kind of modification into a school IEP."

Sister Johnelle Howanach and Melissa Clark

When I first saw Lissie, she looked like the little kids in the Campbell's Soup ads. She had on a sweat shirt and jeans, and shoes that were too big. She came into my house just like she owned the world, her little brown eyes laughing. I didn't know the poor little kid was practically blind—just thought she was the cutest little thing in the whole world.

—JOHNELLE HOWANACH, ON MEETING
SIX-YEAR-OLD MELISSA CLARK IN 1982

One August afternoon in 1982, Johnelle Howanach first met six-year-old "Lissie" Clark. A teaching sister, Johnelle had taken leave from her order to look after her ill parents, who had since died. Staying in the family home in Belt, Montana, she was waiting to have her mother's will probated, and had decided to try foster care until she could return to work. Within days of applying, she received a call from a social worker. Would she consider giving short-term care to a little girl who had been adopted for four years and given back to the authorities because of learning and behaviour problems?

When Lissie arrived for her first visit, she and Johnelle took to each other immediately. They played with Johnelle's hamster and some play-dough that Johnelle whipped up. Lissie had to stay overnight, and before leaving, the social workers warned Johnelle: "They said 'Okay, lady, if you have any thoughts about educating this youngster, forget it, because she is not teachable.'" Johnelle kept quiet, although she "didn't like the idea of anybody saying a child is hopeless. I kind of pride myself that I can teach anybody. You just have to figure out how."

The next morning, after the social workers had taken Lissie back to the emergency foster home, Johnelle made a discovery that might have angered other women. Left-handed Melissa had found a pair of huge right-handed shears, hidden in a drawer. Then she'd cut little half-circles all over her pillowcase. "I never saw her take the shears, never saw her cut with them or put them back. I thought, 'Nobody is going to tell me that a little kid that can do all of this cannot learn.'" And so Lissie became part of her life, because "she was so cute that she stole my heart."

Johnelle learned that her new foster daughter had been born prematurely in 1976, with congenital heart disease, microcephaly and "failure to thrive." As a toddler, she was also diagnosed with severe vision impairment (legal blindness), was speech-delayed, was diagnosed with ADHD, and was one of the first people diagnosed with FAS in Montana.

When Melissa moved into Johnelle's home in Belt, her new foster mother quickly discovered that the little girl was on enough prescription medications for hyperactivity and so-called "seizures" to knock out a horse. She'd been put in hospital because of overdose—she'd gone into a coma—and this was when her adoptive mother had given up. Johnelle told a friend, a nurse, what the dosages were, and was told, "You must be mistaken. She would have to be a giant for them to be giving her that amount." The friend told Johnelle that the high doses of medication could have caused additional brain damage. With a doctor's help, Johnelle began a program of reducing medications—discovering that the drugs had actually *increased* Lissie's hyperactivity. Lissie has not used medications in years.

Johnelle loves to tell the "M story"—an event that took place just before Lissie's seventh birthday. Still in kindergarten, Lissie could not yet read. "The sun was shining through the window and it made the shadow of an M on the carpet." Johnelle ran and got Lissie, took her hand and traced over the "M for Melissa." "I had my hand over hers, tracing the M, and pretty soon I took my hand off and she kept right on, saying 'M, this is my M.' I knew from the look on her face that she knew that was the 'M' and that made the sound 'mmm.'"

Johnelle was now determined that Lissie was going to get an education. By the time Lissie was in third grade, Johnelle spent most evenings working with Lissie, who never complained. With part-time special education and Johnelle's help, Lissie managed to keep up in class, although at the bottom of every subject. "But in math, she wasn't even on the chart."

As children proceed in school, school subjects become more and more abstract, and children with FASD experience increasing difficulty in learning. By seventh grade, things were beginning to fall apart. Teachers and people in the community were advising Johnelle "that I was too over-protective and that I should cut the cord"—words familiar to parents of children with FASD. Despite her gut anxiety, Johnelle allowed Lissie to go to an out-of-town youth conference, as organizers had promised that the event would be "wonderfully chaperoned." Unfortunately, security was poor, and Lissie impulsively "lifted" money from a few tote bags. Everyone knew whom to blame.

The teachers and counsellors failed to understand that this behaviour resulted from Lissie's neurological disabilities when under stress. Lissie's classmates shut her out as well. Because of the community's unsupportive atmosphere, Johnelle and Lissie moved to Great Falls, twenty miles away. Lissie attended a middle school with an excellent program for learning disabled youngsters, and Johnelle worked at an agency for the developmentally disabled.

But when Lissie entered high school, she seemed set up for failure.

Normal high school activities such as learning a locker combination and moving from classroom to classroom, and worst of all the increased independence of high school, were too advanced for Lissie's mental and emotional age. She did well in swimming, and learned to play the flute, but began to skip school, which in youngsters with FASD is generally a sign that the work is becoming too hard. Lissie was placed in a self-contained special education classroom in another school, but the teachers never understood the memory and organizational problems that were a result of from neurological damage.

"I could not get the teachers to write things down for her," says Johnelle. "They said she had to learn to be responsible." Still, Lissie was a talented violinist; she played in the school's string ensemble, and frequently performs solos to this day. With Johnelle's constant support, she graduated from high school in 1996, and then attended a two-year "secondary life skills" program at a nearby college, where she blossomed. "She was reading a lot and her English was just great—she was inquisitive and wanted to learn."

The six-year-old who stole Sister Johnelle's heart is now in her mid-twenties, a talented young woman who plays the violin, sings and has developed a small business marketing gourmet dog foods at the market in Great Falls, Montana. The photo on Lissie's "LuvYum" doggy treats web page (www.lissiesluvyums.com) shows an attractive young woman in horn-rimmed glasses, wearing a beautiful Native American "ribbon dress." After Lissie had tried some jobs that didn't work out, mother and daughter started a small dog-walking service. At Christmas, as gifts for their clients, they baked heart-shaped dog biscuits, stuffed them into pretty teacups and added a gourmet teabag to each saucer. To their astonishment, their clients ordered the biscuits for dog-loving friends, and Johnelle and Lissie suddenly found themselves baking hundreds of dog biscuits each week. They now sell various vacuum-sealed packages—all carrying a message about FASD prevention.

Johnelle and Lissie also speak frequently about FASD at conferences and workshops; Lissie has explored her American Indian roots in the Gros Ventre Assiniboine tribe at Fort Belknap, Montana. Honoured by her tribe for her work in building awareness of FASD, Melissa has been given the name *Eya Be Washday Weya* ("Good Words Woman").

I heard about Melissa and Johnelle ("the most hugged people at the conference") from Dr. Robert Schacht, a professor from Arizona who had written about their amazing presentation on his trip to an Indian reserve in Montana:

> "Lissie" talked about her journey with FAS. She speaks herself, aided by note cards kept in sequence by a metal ring . . . [and] coached from the sidelines by her Mom. . . . She ended her presentation by playing "You are My Sunshine" and "Edelweiss" on the violin. Mother sang the words along with her, and everyone chimed in on the chorus. . . . "Edelweiss" took on new meaning: "Bless my homeland forever" became a reference to Lissie's American Indian reservation. There was scarcely a dry eye in the room.

Lissie also made contact with her biological brother, Melvin Mountain. Unfortunately, Melvin was raised by a foster family who did not understand that his many problems were related to prenatal alcohol. Frequently in trouble with the law, he "did not get the help and support that he needed," says Johnelle. Despite the best efforts of Johnelle and Melissa, he committed suicide on Good Friday, 2002, at the age of twenty-one. "Neither of us realized how bad his pain was," says Johnelle.

Johnelle, in her late sixties, worries about what will happen when she's too old to be Melissa's "external forebrain." Who else could ever be so accepting, so understanding of Melissa's disabilities? "She is the sweetest, kindest, most inquisitive person," says Johnelle. "There is nothing about her that I don't absolutely love."

The Gelo Clan

What kind of people would be insane enough to take on seven alcohol-affected children? And what kind of woman would *voluntarily* load all

253

seven of these children, ranging in age from fifteen months to sixteen years, into a Chevy Astro Van for a month-long trip? Julie Gelo drove her charges across the United States and back, and wrote a warm and funny article about her survival strategies:

> Each child had a Walkman or CD player with headset and a selection
> of tapes, plus we had snacks and one whole box filled with travel toys.
> The night before we left, I bathed everyone and dressed them in com-
> fortable shorts. All their shoes were lined up at the front door. My
> goal was to have everyone loaded and be heading out the driveway by
> 6:30 a.m., and we were only about ten minutes late. (Julie Gelo, "How
> I Spent My Summer Vacation," *Iceberg,* March 2001)

Julie and her husband, Lynn, live in Bothell, Washington, just outside Seattle. They are among the several families I know who have voluntarily taken on a number of alcohol-affected children. Julie explains that "We never intended to do anything permanent—we were only going to do our bit for society." The seven youngsters are now there permanently—the couple have adopted four of the children and are permanent guardians of the other three.

Married in 1988, both for the second time, Julie and Lynn had a huge blended family *without* their transplanted children. Julie has three adult daughters and five grandchildren by her first marriage. Lynn has an adult son and daughter and two grandchildren by his first marriage; his second daughter, Tari, contracted encephalitis as a toddler, and died at age twenty.

Until 1993 Julie had never heard the term "fetal alcohol syndrome," although it had been defined two decades earlier by University of Washington researchers. At that time, she and Lynn were fostering two teenaged Samoan boys. "None of our parenting skills with our other six kids were working." Then Julie's daughter, Jessica, a high school senior, brought home a huge packet of papers that she had been given by a woman who spoke about FAS at her school. Julie read the literature and instantly recognized what she'd been dealing with. Calling the boys' case worker, she asked if their mother had drunk during pregnancy, and was told there was a high likelihood that she had. When Julie asked if the boys had ever been assessed for FAS, the case worker had never heard of it.

After reading Michael Dorris's book *The Broken Cord,* Julie immediately made an appointment with Dr. Sterling Clarren at the University of Washington's diagnostic clinic. However, Julie had no baby photos and could not confirm that the boys' birth mother had drunk alcohol while pregnant. Small size is often a tip-off to FAS, but as the boys were Samoan they were exceptionally large—one of them weighed 335 pounds. Consequently, despite their learning and behaviour problems, the clinic could not diagnose FAS. "We did get a diagnosis of neurological impairment. They just couldn't tell us if it was because of the alcohol or because they had been disciplined by getting hit in the head with a baseball bat."

Julie and Lynn had a huge house, and when the Samoan boys left, the couple decided to try doing foster care with younger children who "wouldn't steal our car and get into drugs." They heard of the great need for foster parents for Native American children, but were told by the Indian Unit that, as Caucasians, they would not be able to keep any foster children permanently. Julie and Lynn understood perfectly, but the children are still there.

It's a complicated web of relationships. Theadore (born in 1984), Ricky (1991) and Nickolaus (1994) are biological brothers. Michael (1989) and Tessa (1999), of Canadian aboriginal background, have the same birth mother. Brandan (1995) and Cayenne (1999), of Northern Cheyenne heritage, are first cousins. Julie and Lynn have been allowed to adopt Michael, Tessa, Brandon and Cayenne, and are permanent guardians of brothers Theadore, Ricky and Nickolaus.

Julie's description of the damage done to her children is heartbreaking. Tessa, with an IQ between 106 and 110, is the brightest but most damaged. Exposed prenatally to alcohol and cocaine, she was held on a heater in infancy and suffered third-degree burns. She has been diagnosed with post traumatic stress disorder. Despite her good verbal skills and cute personality, she has learning disabilities in written language and math, and is extremely anxious. Because Tessa's many learning and emotional problems are invisible, Julie finds it difficult to obtain services for her.

Julie had been a mentor to "Alice," birth mother of Theodore, Ricky and Nickolaus. Alice, who has FASD herself, has given birth to six alcohol-affected children, and her oldest daughter has also given birth to a baby with FASD. "So we're into the third generation of alcohol-affected infants," says Julie. (At $2 million for the lifetime costs of each of these eight people—Alice, her six children and one grandchild—we're looking at a family who will cost U.S. taxpayers a total of $16 million.)

Nickolaus, at seven the youngest of Alice's children, has been with the Gelos since the age of eleven months, and is the most damaged of the three siblings. Normal in size, he has the facial features of FAS, and a CAT scan has indicated a hole in the brain near his left temple. He's in a highly structured, low-stimulus classroom with seven other children, taught by four adults.

Brandan was diagnosed with full FAS at three and a half months. Julie brought him home from the neonatal intensive care unit when he was ten days old, and he needed a feeding tube for the first year of his life. Unable to suck or swallow, he suffered from pneumonia and ear infections, and doctors told the Gelos that he probably wouldn't live to his first birthday. A neurologist told Julie that Brandan would likely be so mentally damaged that he would not respond to people, and would have to be institutionalized. Tiny, he is microcephalic (has a small head), has an IQ of 64 and has all the facial features of FAS.

In 1999 a worker with Brandan's Northern Cheyenne tribe called Julie to say that Brandan had a first cousin, a baby girl named Cayenne—would the Gelos be interested in adopting her? This request was highly unusual, as in both the U.S. and Canada non-natives are generally not allowed to adopt native children. Earlier, tribal officials had also decided that the Gelos could offer the best permanent home for Tessa and Michael.

"That has been a great honour and gift to us," says Julie. "The trust that the tribal community has put in us doesn't happen very often." Cayenne's name reflects her temperament. Exposed prenatally to alcohol, cocaine and heroin, she suffered from morphine withdrawal for the first four weeks of her life. Tiny, without the facial features of FAS, she is delayed in language, but can carry out directions, something Julie's other children have had difficulty doing.

When Brandan, aged three and a half months, was diagnosed by the Clarren clinic in 1995, he was the tenth child that Julie had taken for a diagnosis. [She had previously taken the two Samoan boys, her six foster and adoptive children, and a foster child who had come and gone.] She approached Doctors Sterling Clarren and Susan Astley with a suggestion. "I felt that they needed to have a parent on their team— someone who lives with FAS on a daily basis." To her surprise, they asked her to take on the job. Since that time, she has been the clinic's family advocate, attends clinics every Friday, is present when children are diagnosed and presents frequently at conferences across North America. When Astley and Clarren train diagnostic teams, they now insist that a family advocate be part of that team.

By 1996 Julie, familiar with the symptoms of fetal alcohol syndrome, began wondering about her biological daughter Faith, then twenty-five and living in Minnesota. Faith had completed her high school diploma, but school had been far more difficult for her than for younger sisters Jessica and Brianna. "As she got older, she had more problems with peer groups, and didn't understand social innuendo." As an older adolescent and young adult, Faith had made some poor choices about relationships, and had great difficulty understanding time and money, frequently bouncing rent checks or being overdrawn at the bank.

Faith was tiny, six inches shorter than her younger sisters. "I pulled out her baby pictures and looked at them. She looked like Brandan, except she was blond and blue-eyed and Brandan had black hair and black eyes." Julie, an alcoholic in recovery, tried to remember how much she was drinking as a teenager. Faith had been born two days after Julie's eighteenth birthday, in 1972—one year before FAS had been officially defined. Julie remembered how she had binge-drunk right up to the end of her fifth month of pregnancy.

Faith was by now married and pregnant herself. Julie took the photos of her daughter to Dr. Sterling Clarren. During Faith's next visit, Clarren diagnosed her with full-blown FAS. Even after sixteen years of sobriety, Julie was devastated. "I really thought that I had asked forgiveness of everybody that my drinking had harmed. Then I had to come to grips with the fact that the person I had harmed the most was my own child."

Sobbing, Julie tried to apologize to Faith, who put her arms around her mother, and with the usual FAS generosity of spirit said, "Mom, it's okay. I know that you didn't do it because you wanted to hurt me—you just didn't know any better. I'm just glad to know that I'm not stupid."

Julie says that doing foster care was the best possible means of teaching birth control and alcohol abstinence to her birth daughters. "None of my daughters had teen pregnancies, none of my grandchildren is alcohol-exposed." Like Julie, her husband, Lynn, has been in recovery for many years, and both parents have worked hard at educating their adoptive and foster children about alcohol. Julie tells them, "Alcohol and drugs are poison to you guys, just like they are poison to me, and poison to Dad."

> Brandan came home from kindergarten one day last year, and they'd had a visitor, talking about alcohol, drugs and tobacco. He came home and he said, "Smoking is bad for you, isn't it, Mom?" And I said yes, it is. He said, "I can't ever drink and do drugs?" And I said, that's right, you can't ever drink and do drugs. He said, "Because it is illegal, and I would be unarrested."
>
> I said, you betcha, Brandan—you would be unarrested!

Common Denominators

Almost all of the birth and adoptive parents I've encountered, and many of the "temporary" foster parents, have a deep and abiding love for their children, and will fight for them like a mother lion will fight for her cubs. But the Superparents seem to resemble those inflatable punching clown toys: they bounce back smiling after adversity, while the rest of us begin to wilt after one punch too many. What, then, makes the difference?

I've observed that the parents of "marvel" kids with FASD seem to have remarkable abilities that go further than those universal protective factors outlined in the secondary disabilities study. (The six key factors that protect against secondary disabilities are 1) a stable, nurturing household, 2) diagnosis under age six, 3) no violence experienced, 4) staying in each home for three or more years, 5) quality of home environment between eight and twelve, and 6) diagnosis of FAS rather than FAE.)

It helps if the main caregiver has a loving, equally committed partner who can take over from time to time, and if the community environment supports the entire family. But many of the Superparents are raising their children alone, without much community support. Here are some common characteristics I've noticed in the parents interviewed for this chapter and other Superparents: total acceptance, knowledge, reduced expectations, commitment, creativity, a positive outlook, and—possibly most important—a whopping sense of humour.

Accepting the Roller Coaster

Marceil "Marcy" Ten Eyck, a Seattle therapist, has such a complicated blended family that I had to map it out on a sheet of paper during our phone interview. Between them, she and her husband, Jim Fox, have seven adult children, related by birth, adoption or marriage—including three alcohol-affected daughters and a son with severe cerebral palsy. Marcy's two biological adult daughters were diagnosed with FASD—one as an adolescent, the other as an adult—and Marcy is proud that both are leading normal lives, although each young woman has faced many challenges in her lifetime.

As a parent and therapist, Marcy has come to believe that the grief process in coming to accept that a child has FASD can often be harder than dealing with more obvious physical or mental disabilities, terminal illness or even death. The latter situations seem more tragic, but the parent moves through the stages of denial, bargaining, anger, sadness and finally, acceptance, and is able to move on.

> But with fetal alcohol, in my experience, one day things are terrible: we are floating between anger and frustration and sobbing. A day later this person can be an absolute delight, and all of a sudden we are back into denial. We are up and down in the grief process, and yes, we do finally get to acceptance, but three days later you might be back into denial. You have to accept the roller coaster. (Marceil Ten Eyck, interview with author)

Teresa Kellerman told me of her years of chronic "heavy-duty grief." Like many adoptive parents, she at first was furious with John's birth mother: *How could she do this to an innocent baby?* Then she realized that John's first mother was a victim too: she had grown up in an alcoholic family, was introduced to alcohol at an early age, had likely been physically and/or sexually abused and might have been alcohol-affected herself. "So my anger eventually took on different targets— the teachers who didn't know how to teach him, the doctors who didn't know how to treat him, the social workers and psychologists who didn't understand him."

Some parents never get to the grief process because they don't know what they're dealing with. Marcy Ten Eyck's biological daughter Sydney was not diagnosed with fetal alcohol syndrome until age fourteen. Marcy later learned that baby Sydney had been passed over by the University of Washington doctors who made the original study of fetal alcohol syndrome. "If you see her baby pictures, you can see all of the FAS features. But her mother was a Girl Scout executive and her father was a special investigative agent. Nobody thought to ask me if I'd had a drink—and I was pretty much into the late stage of alcoholism!"

My own process of accepting Colette's fetal alcohol damage took five years, from the time my friend Keitha, a recovering alcoholic, suggested that my daughter's learning and behaviour problems could have been caused by her birth mother's alcoholism. It was easier to believe that the tantrums and learning difficulties were the result of being adopted at three, and that if we could find the right therapist, everything would be fine. Like Julie Gelo and Marcy Ten Eyck, many birth mothers of alcohol-affected children struggle with denial even longer than I did, particularly if they don't fit the stereotype of poorly educated alcoholic women in poverty.

Many adoptive fathers have difficulty accepting the possibility of fetal alcohol damage, and believe that, in seeking a diagnosis, their wives are giving their children "an excuse for bad behaviour." I've seen several instances in which an adoptive mother has tracked down family histories that indicate alcoholic birth parents, and taken articles, brochures, videos and books about FASD to her husband. Nevertheless, the father would prefer to throw the child out than consider that he is not really evil, lazy or stupid, but struggling with neurological damage. The mother is torn between her husband and her child, and in many cases the marriage breaks up as a result.

Marcy Ten Eyck and Donna Debolt both believe that grief therapy can be extremely helpful in allowing parents of children with FASD to move on, and help their children and themselves. Donna outlines the long list of losses that can flatten birth, adoptive or long-term foster parents as they come to terms with their child's disabilities:

- hopes and dreams for the child;
- self-esteem and confidence;
- a balanced family system;
- support from family and friends;
- financial security;
- privacy;
- freedom (we're often held hostage by our children with FASD, because no one will babysit them); and
- ability to share in accomplishments.

Worst of all, parents of alcohol-affected children may lose the child through separation, adoption breakdown, running away, or even death.

All of the parents interviewed for this chapter have learned to focus on their children's strengths rather than their weaknesses. At some point, they stopped being embarrassed by their children's behaviour, stopped caring how the community views them or their children, learned to ignore well-meaning friends, family and professionals who advised them to "back off" and let their children sink in order to "teach them responsibility." They stopped railing at the "system," and began to forge alliances with others who shared their goals. Nurtured by a supportive community—even if it consisted only of online friends—they even learned to laugh at many problems that earlier made them cry.

There are no short cuts on the journey through grief. But when we parents stop raging at our children and at the community's lack of support; when we begin to view our children as whole and perfect regardless of their disabilities; when we become their allies rather than their adversaries; when we talk about their problems openly; when we begin to help other families work for change—then miracles happen.

Our children begin to heal, and so do we.

CHAPTER FOURTEEN

The Spinning Kaleidoscope

*While you'd think that someone with such an addictive past—
crack, coke, pot—would turn to booze, I don't know why I didn't
drink while on the streets. When I got pregnant with my son, I
had a roof over my head, and the first thing I remember was
that my dad and mother and their friends were not too happy
about my pregnancy. They thought I would drink and use drugs.
Well, I proved them so wrong.*

—COLETTE AT TWENTY-THREE, SPEAKING AT
A CONFERENCE ON FASD, APRIL 2003

We were tempted to be smug. In the six years between 1997 and 2003,
we'd learned a lot. We now knew that a diagnosis of prenatal alcohol
damage before the child is six is a key factor in preventing problems in
adulthood, yet Colette, who had not been diagnosed with ARND until
eighteen, was managing well. She drank no alcohol in pregnancy; we
adored her little brown-eyed son and strawberry-blond daughter, and
enjoyed a good relationship with her. Some members of our online support groups thought we were "Superparents." I felt I had to point out that
our family's "success" was as vulnerable as a glass house in a hailstorm.

Colette's life was not easy, but with her usual stoicism, she rarely
complained. Her partner also had learning disabilities that limited

employment possibilities. For five years, they lived on her small Ontario Disability Support cheques: if they jointly earned more than a few hundred dollars, the provincial government would claw back their benefits. As trustee of her disability support, Brian ensured that rent and utilities were paid.

Ever since our grandchildren were born, we had been concerned that their parents could not give them the material things that middle-class children take for granted, and we'd tried to fill in the gaps. Colette and her partner were likely to live permanently on social services, always be underhoused and never be able to never afford a car or lessons in sports, dance or music. They would have difficulty dealing with the children's teachers or helping with homework. But our greatest fear was that schools and the community would fail these bright, beautiful children, just as they had failed their parents.

In trying to help Colette, we'd realized that the public knew next to nothing about the size and scope of FASD, and by 1998 we had become determined to use our skills as communicators to get the message out. We changed our lives accordingly. We downsized from our big old house to a suburban California-style home, perfect for empty nesters, and sold our country property. Needing proper office space with room to accommodate the books, papers and files of our volunteer work, we purchased a building in Toronto's Greek community.

Many parents describe the FASD experience as a roller coaster, but to me it has been a constantly spinning kaleidoscope, with an endless series of designs and patterns. By early 2003 Colette was fed up with living in poverty, and she enrolled in an adult learning centre where she could complete her remaining high school credits with just one co-op course. Her decision set our family's kaleidoscope spinning again. Colette's long, often difficult relationship with her children's father ended. Nearly five years of pregnancy and parenting small children in poverty, beginning when she was nineteen, had robbed her of much of her youth, and she was mentally and physically exhausted.

The co-op course gave her a taste of the possibilities she had missed. At twenty-four, but emotionally still in her teens, she is attempting to figure out just who she is. Knowing she was unable to parent adequately, she asked for our help, and currently her little son and daughter are living with us. Like the alcohol-affected daughters of many of our colleagues, she has now struggled with every single secondary disability, including separation from her children. I keep wondering if anything could have prevented this sad design.

Could This Family Have Been Saved?

We've been told that "Harriet," Colette's birth mother, was twelve when she was abandoned by an alcoholic mother. Her father, who raised her, was also addicted to alcohol, and Harriet soon began to drink too. Binge-drinking through each pregnancy, Harriet gave birth to three children; Colette was the third. All of them were removed from her care at the same time. When sober, she was a devoted, gentle, responsible mother; the loss of her children was a devastating blow that drove her even further into addiction. I now believe that Harriet was a "stack attack victim," damaged by prenatal alcohol, then abused and neglected as a child.

If Harriet had been helped by an outreach program such as P-CAP at the University of Washington or Toronto's Breaking the Cycle after her first child was born—or even better, during her first pregnancy—Colette's brain could have been spared the insult of alcohol. Free long-term residential treatment for *both* parents, along with the children, before Colette was even conceived, might have enabled both parents to sober up and raise her. Given her intelligence and abilities with animals, Colette might have been studying veterinary medicine by now.

Possibly only a minority of addicted couples could be helped by residential programs, if they existed. But even if only 10 percent of these families were saved, fewer damaged babies would be born, fewer youngsters would be traumatized by being removed from biological parents and governments would be spared the expense of foster care for thousands of children. More investment in supporting addicted parents during pregnancy and afterwards would reduce harm to babies and save society countless dollars.

Forever Families

Currently, tens of thousands of foster children across North America, ranging in age from toddlers to teenagers, need permanent homes. Many have been exposed to prenatal alcohol, but may also be as bright and engaging as Colette. Each of these children needs a "forever family"—loving people who will understand his disabilities and be his lifelong advocates. How ironic that countless infertile couples are seeking perfect new babies, either through private adoption or fertility treatments such as in vitro fertilization, when so many "older" children (over the age of one year) need loving permanent homes. Most prospective parents run when they hear the words "fetal alcohol." But two decades ago, few families would consider adopting a child with Down syndrome. Today, many adoptive parents are delighted with their sweet youngsters with Down syndrome, knowing that early intervention can boost their abilities.

In my observation, around half of all children adopted in the past two decades seem to have been affected to some degree by fetal alcohol, but few have been diagnosed. Rates of FASD among adopted children of aboriginal, African-American and Eastern European background may be even higher. Donna Debolt's southern Alberta figures indicate that about 70 percent of children available for adoption through child protection agencies have some degree of FASD, and this percentage is likely similar nationally. If all children entering the foster care system were screened for FASD and given adequate support—emotional, educational, financial and medical—for the rest of their lives, industrialized societies could head off countless expensive tragedies. If the Children's Aid Society had warned us that Colette might have fetal alcohol damage, just as they had warned us that Cleo might have inherited a tendency towards depression, Brian and I could have been much more effective parents.

Every year, about 327,000 babies are born in Canada, and Ann Streissguth and others believe that about 2 in 1,000—around 650 Canadian infants annually—will have full FAS.[52] Another, much larger group—around 2,000—will have the subtle neurological damage of pFAS or ARND. Of the 4 million babies born annually in the U.S., around 8,000 are likely to have full FAS and another 30,000 will have pFAS or ARND.[53] Only those with obvious physical or mental defects will be correctly diagnosed. The rest will struggle through life, experiencing difficulties in school, the job market and human relationships—and neither they nor their families will understand why they just can't "get it."

In Canada, about 20,000 permanent wards of the government are living in foster homes, waiting and hoping for a "forever family." In the U.S., about 100,000 foster children are available for adoption, most with histories of neglect and abuse. Because alcohol is almost always involved in the family breakdown, they are at high risk of the secondary disabilities of FASD. Without loving, knowledgable, determined, *permanent* families, they are doomed to repeat their parents' life scripts.

Elspeth Ross, co-facilitator of the Fetal Alcohol Syndrome Association of Ottawa, board member of the Adoption Council of Canada and parent of two sons with FASD, is a passionate spokesperson for adoption. Her determined older son, now married, is a college graduate, and her younger son is still at home. "People seem afraid to talk about FASD, as if it is some horrible thing . . . [but] we should be more willing to talk about it, and say, 'Yeah, this is a possibility, but it's not the end of the world—some of us are managing.'"

Elspeth says that parents need to be informed about FASD, and educated about what the "norms" are. (I wish that Brian and I had better understood Colette's habit of "borrowing.") Parents of alcohol-affected children generally won't get adequate understanding from family and friends, she says. They will need to seek it out from other FASD-affected families, support groups, electronic mail-lists, conferences and the few professionals who understand the disorder. "You need referrals to the right services—but many people aren't getting them." And finally, she says, what the adoptive family needs is the commitment "to hang in with your kids no matter how hard it is."

Ann Streissguth's research indicates that as many as 80 percent of alcohol-affected children are not raised by their families of origin.[54] Since I saw that TV show in March 1997, I have communicated with hundreds of parents and caregivers of children with FASD—birth, foster, adoptive, stepparents, extended family—and most feel that they have been let down by friends, family, neighbours, schools, professionals, governments and adoption agencies. Friends and family often view parents of children with FASD as "enabling." Neighbours get fed up with out-of-control youngsters who may lie, steal and throw tantrums. Schools often ignore diagnoses and parents' pleas for strategies and programs geared to their children's needs. Doctors, psychologists, psychiatrists and social workers, often ignorant of the complexity of FASD, may fail to recognize the symptoms and, as a result, give inappropriate therapy or advice.

Parents are crushed under bills for medication, tutoring, special camps and private schools. In recent years, the federal governments of both Canada and the U.S. have put many millions of dollars into strategies relating to FASD; however, most of this money has funded projects for salaried professionals. Almost none has gone to help the families who are raising these kids. When the community fails to support FASD families, they are at high risk of breaking down, and then everybody pays: affected children, parents and society at large.

What does it feel like to be a child who is removed from his biological family, and later abandoned by foster or adoptive parents? Even with impaired learning, you learn not to trust and may become incapable of forming deep relationships. Every time a child is moved to a different home, she becomes less able to attach, more likely to become a "stack attack victim." Prospective adoptive and foster parents should know that in order to flourish these beautiful and often delightful youngsters will need exceptional parents—people with huge hearts, good mental and physical health, determination, commitment and a wacky sense of humour. Agencies must invest in teaching families about FASD before they adopt. Just knowing that your child's sometimes-odd behaviour is related to neurological problems could reduce anxiety and blaming. (If Brian and I had known that the mess in Colette's room was caused by too many possessions, we could have eliminated both the clutter and the nagging.)

What Families Need

Donna Debolt and Mary Berube, Alberta social workers specializing in FASD, have developed a simple document outlining the needs of families living with affected children. Mary Berube also has two adult sons with FASD: her younger son is featured in Canada's National Film Board documentary *David with FAS*.

The Debolt/Berube paper, "Guidelines to Intervention in Families," outlines how social workers can best meet the needs of the various kinds of families in the fetal alcohol spectrum. Nearly all adoptive and foster families would be classified as "Unaffected Adult Caring for Affected Children." The description of the "unaffected adult" dealing with the child with FASD resonates with Mary's experience as a mother. The authors describe the parent as reporting "high frustration, exhaustion, isolation and depression." He uses crisis language, may say "crazy things" and may want the child or children out of the home. The parent may also have problems with adult relationships, lose his sense of humour, say that "nothing works" and claim that previous attempts to find help were useless or damaging. He may be in financial crisis, and may have developed addictions that need to be assessed (in my case, chocolate chip cookies).

Key things that the unaffected adult needs are

- ongoing education about FASD in order to learn caregiving strategies and understand the behaviours of children affected by prenatal alcohol;
- support before and through her child's diagnosis, and ongoing support afterwards;

- therapy for grieving and loss;
- connections with other caregivers;
- a case manager;
- [and my favourite:] *respite even when not asked for* (rarely available in most parts of the world).

Debolt and Berube also outline the needs of children with FASD—support they rarely receive, support that all of us should be fighting for. They need

- early diagnosis of FASD, followed by assessment of strengths and limitations;
- a protected environment, increased supervision and structure (i.e., SCREAMS);
- a supportive family who understand their disabilities; and
- a management team, which could include professionals in medicine, speech/language, education, skill-building, and behaviour management *focused on prevention of behaviours.* (We can't change the child; we have to figure out a way to change the environment.)

I'd like to add another need: *financial assistance.* Nearly every family of FASD children is desperately short of cash because of the youngsters' many special needs.

Debolt and Berube also look at the presentation and needs of the "affected adult caring for the unaffected child," and "affected adult caring for the affected child." I take comfort in their statement that unaffected children whose parents have FASD often display "amazing strengths." We've observed these qualities in our own two small grandchildren—emotionally hurting, yet as valiant and tender as Hansel and Gretel.

Judging by the experience of families I know all over the world, the needs of children with FASD and their parents are almost never met. Yet investing in FASD families would go a long way towards preventing parental burnout. It would keep families together, reduce the number of alcohol-affected adolescents who drop out of school and wind up on the street and alleviate expensive social problems such as poverty, homelessness and crime.

Readin' and 'Ritin' and 'Rithmatic

Despite her many years of special education, the school system let Colette down for two reasons. First, she had never been diagnosed with a fetal alcohol disorder. Second, even if she had been diagnosed, the resources to teach her were not in place. Children with FASD need

- knowledgable, creative, compassionate teachers and principals;
- simple, bare classrooms free of distractions;
- very small classes, specific to their needs;
- a curriculum that understands their poor memories, and breaks down learning into very small segments, repeating each segment over and over again;
- a concrete, hands-on approach to learning; and
- recognition and understanding of their behaviour problems. (For many children with FASD, the hardest subjects are *lunch* and *recess,* times when they repeatedly get into trouble.)

Children with FASD generally can't concentrate for an extended period of time. Many will learn best in the morning, and do better if they can have subjects such as physical education, art and music in the afternoon. An inventive teacher can use these activities to provide learning opportunities that will help with more academic subjects (e.g., using softball to teach math).

Math is nearly always a problem for youngsters with FASD. I'd suggest they be taught to use calculators for everyday math problems, such as shopping for groceries. For youngsters with FASD, advanced math and foreign languages should not be mandatory for graduation from high school. If a youngster had deformed feet and was unable to run, would we force him to pass physical education in order to graduate?

Children and adolescents with FASD have difficulty following through on term projects without considerable supervision. I spent countless hours helping both of my daughters with class projects, generally when they began weeping the night before the project was due. In fact, I think homework should be abolished for youngsters with FASD. They have great difficulty working independently, and by evening they're too burned out to do any more work—just as you are at the end of the day.

Diagnosis: Key to Understanding

Identification is the first step. Parents, caregivers and school communities that understand the child can work around his weaknesses, build on his strengths and preserve his self-esteem. Unfortunately, many children are never diagnosed because of the shame and blame felt by most mothers who drank any amount at all in pregnancy. Here are some other reasons why a child or adult with FASD might never be diagnosed:

- She is adopted, and the birth information regarding maternal drinking is not available.
- He is a foster child, and overworked agency staff are too preoccupied with finding homes for the children in care, and heading off disasters, to concentrate on one child's condition.
- She is the child of a middle-class or wealthy woman. No doctor has ever asked the mother, "Did you drink in pregnancy?" The child has been diagnosed with attention deficit hyperactivity disorder, or another mental health disorder.
- The mother is a light or moderate drinker, who may have had four or five drinks on a few social occasions in early pregnancy, but did not drink after she realized she was pregnant.

- The child's doctor is unaware that prenatal alcohol damage to the central nervous system can occur without the small head, small size, flat philtrum, and short palpebral fissures (eye slits) that signal full-blown FAS.
- The child, adolescent or adult may have excellent verbal strengths and seeming insight. As one psychologist puts it, "He can talk as if he's really thinking things through."
- Her doctor believes that there is no point in getting a diagnosis, because brain damage is permanent and nothing can be done to help anyway, so why label this person?
- He has a normal IQ: parents, school and doctors believe that his learning and behaviour problems are the result of laziness and unwillingness to pay attention.
- She lives in an isolated community, without access to a diagnostic clinic.
- He lives in a big city, but there are no well-trained diagnosticians there.

But even a youngster or adult who has received a diagnosis may not be fully understood. Her behaviour may infuriate family members and others in the community: her teacher, social worker, employer, lawyer, probation officer or peers. Okay, she has neurological damage, but why won't she tell the truth, stop stealing, do what she's asked to do or follow through on her promises? Many people she encounters don't understand that her so-called "acting out" is actually part of her disability.

When we fail to understand children with FASD, they are likely to become failed adolescents and adults, unemployed, addicted, possibly homeless or in trouble with the law. Because few of those thousands of people with FASD who are homeless or in the prison system are ever diagnosed, they receive little informed support. Professionals and the public often view them as "bad," and alcohol-affected people often don't mind this perception. Allan Mountford, a special education teacher in Ontario's Durham Region, explains, "A person with FASD would often rather appear 'tough' than stupid."

What Adults with FASD Need

Over the past thirty years, researchers have developed numerous strategies that can help individuals with FASD. Most will never be able to live independently; they will always need that external brain. Donna Debolt calls external brain people "do-fers."

Employment Training and Support

Older adolescents and adults need vocational training, job coaches and employers willing to take on the challenge of this complex disability. An employee with FASD needs ongoing training, a structured environment, checklists, repetition, reminders, good role models and recognition by staff that his problems are caused by neurological impairment. Supervision is key: Colette spent several months working in an entry-level position in which every other staff member gave her orders. Before she had completed one task, someone would interrupt with another menial request. She generally lost track of what she was supposed to be doing, was rebuked for failing to follow through and eventually lost the job. Her experience is all too common.

Supported Income and Housing

Adults with FASD need permanent disability pensions that will enable them to work part-time or full-time in low-paying jobs and still live decently; most will need a trustee to ensure that bills get paid. These pensions must include drug and dental plans, as people with FASD often have many health problems. Rather than clawing back earned income and paying social workers to make sure that recipients don't cheat, we should view this pension as justly deserved, and just let them pay income tax.

We must invest in effective, long-term residential housing for those adolescents with FASD whose behaviour makes it impossible for them to live at home, and for adults with FASD, who now make up a significant number of the homeless. Such housing would be far cheaper and more humane than jail, which is where many alcohol-affected youths and adults end up.

Unfortunately, many tenants with FASD tend to be "hard to house" —landlords' nightmares who fail to pay the rent and have great difficulty maintaining tidy premises. When governments invest in subsidized housing for people living in poverty, failing to understand that many have FASD, the buildings often deteriorate into slums. Possibly we should be looking at a kibbutz-type model for people with FASD— a nurturing, structured, well-supervised urban or rural community where sleeping spaces are private, but most other activities, including employment, cooking and eating and child care, are communal.

Effective Birth Control

All women with FASD of childbearing age who are sexually active need free, effective, easily accessible birth control. Depo Provera currently seems to be a good choice as it's non-invasive and a woman requires only four injections per year. She also needs an external brain to ensure that she gets the shots. Colette did well on Depo Provera as long as I took her for those quarterly shots, bribing her with a steak meal afterwards. Then she decided to "take control" of her fertility. Two children later, she did take control—permanently.

Easily Accessible Alcohol and Drug Rehabilitation Programs

If a knowledgable, effective drug treatment program had been available when Colette was fourteen, she and our family might have been spared years of grief. We need free long-term residential alcohol and drug rehabilitation programs for adolescents under the age of 18 (such programs are currently almost nonexistent for young females), and for all women of childbearing age and their partners.

Females with FASD are at high risk of bringing more alcohol-affected children into the world. Unfortunately, twelve-step programs with the abstract concept of the "Higher Power" are often ineffective for addicts with FASD. Talk sessions relying on insight are usually a waste of time: people with FASD often seem insightful, but then repeat their dysfunctional behaviour. Alcohol or drug addicts with FASD generally have difficulty keeping appointments, and need an external brain to ensure they get to their addiction counsellor or twelve-step meeting.

Native North American healing traditions—sweat lodges, healing circles—have been helpful to many addicts of aboriginal background, and similar physical/spiritual treatments might be equally effective for non-natives. I'd like to see a pilot residential program at least four weeks long, in which participants would deal with addictions through practical, healthy, concrete activities such as games, music, art, dance and cooking. Long-term follow-up would be required, and an external brain could ensure they attended sessions after "graduation."

FASD and the Criminal Justice System

Colette's one brush with the law, at fourteen, should have provided an opportunity for intervention. The fact that she was adopted, came from an alcoholic background and was dabbling in soft drugs should have tipped off the judge at her bail hearing. She would have been far better off if, instead of that lengthy court process, he had ordered that she be assessed for FASD, and that appropriate structures be put in place to ensure that she completed school and received help for her addiction problems.

Every person involved with criminal justice, anywhere in the world—police officers, lawyers, judges, prison personnel—should be familiar with the excellent 1998 report *Fetal Alcohol Syndrome: Implications for Correctional Service* commissioned by Correctional

Service Canada (www.csc-scc.gc.ca). The authors recommend that suspected cases of FASD be identified early in the incarceration process,
and suggest pre-sentence screening to determine whether an offender
has ever been assessed for prenatal alcohol damage. They stress the
need for extensive planning for inmates with FASD well before release:
housing, job training, life skills training and *close and supportive monitoring after their return to the community.*

Education and Awareness

No national government anywhere has yet developed a large-scale
media campaign informing citizens about the invisible epidemic of
FASD. As a result, more than three decades after fetal alcohol syndrome
was officially defined, many Canadians still believe that only alcoholic
women can damage their babies, and that these infants are all small,
severely damaged, obviously mentally impaired and probably of native
heritage. The wording of the frequently used message that "alcohol in
pregnancy can hurt your baby," is not strong enough. Every woman of
childbearing age should know the truth; the signs should warn that
"even *small* amounts of prenatal alcohol can permanently affect your
baby's brain."

The public also needs to know that we all encounter people with
undiagnosed FASD every day of our lives: those skinny young women
thumbing rides on the motel strip; the acting-out kids plaguing the
teachers in our local school; the homeless guy sitting on the sidewalk;
and the youth with "ADHD" from the upscale family, who has tried
every drug going. Society views all of these people as losers, rather than
understanding that they share a strange but common disability and will
need extra support as long as they live.

Every doctor, psychiatrist, psychologist, teacher, social worker,
police officer, lawyer, judge, probation officer, politician, journalist
and public servant needs to be well informed about FASD.
Professionals in education, health, legal and social services should

refer clients suspected of FASD for diagnosis, if possible, and make sure that any plan of treatment or care takes into account their probable neurological disabilities.

FASD needs to be on school curricula as part of health and family studies programs. Because at least one percent of children in elementary, middle school and early high school, are living with the effects of prenatal alcohol, such programs need to be taught with the utmost sensitivity. Teachers must take care in explaining a disability that causes young people to have great difficulty in school, exhibit problems in judgment, possibly steal and lie and be unpopular with their peers—when Nathan or Samantha, with all of these problems, is sitting in the classroom.

College and university students also need to be informed about FASD in courses such as biology, psychology and sociology, but also as part of the educational institution's extracurricular activities—the "fun stuff" that so often encourages both alcohol and sex. Young women and men should know that *if they are sexually active and not using effective birth control, they are planning a pregnancy.* They also need to know that any amount of alcohol, any time in pregnancy, can harm the baby.

The Snowstorm Brainstorm

Digging out in the great Toronto snowstorm in January 1999, Brian and I realized that on the ninth day of the ninth month of 1999, a lot of nines would come together. Why not use the opportunity of 9/9/99 to remind the world that during the nine months of pregnancy, alcohol is dangerous to the fetus? We sent a message to our e-mail friends, and within hours Teresa Kellerman, Brian and I were organizing online volunteers, planning the first International FAS Awareness Day, on September 9, 1999, with a Minute of Reflection at 9:09 a.m.

The first FAS Day (now often called FASDay) was observed by volunteers across the U.S. and Canada, and also in New Zealand, the U.K., South Africa and Germany. Among those keen international volunteers were Ann Gibson, Vivien Lourens, Shirley Winikerei and Christine Rogan (introduced in chapter 12), who now spearhead national awareness activities in their own countries. Working with little money, but harnessing creativity, passion and the Internet, volunteers began building knowledge in their own communities, informing the public through countless newspaper, radio and TV items. We did it again in 2000, with even greater success, but in 2001 our volunteers' hard work was overshadowed by the tragedy of September 11 two days later.

FAS Day has been recognized by Health Canada, the U.S. government's Substance Abuse and Mental Health Services Administration (SAMHSA) and many provincial and state governments. Each year, volunteers in a few more countries come on board. In June 2002, the Saskatchewan legislature unanimously passed a bill permanently establishing FAS Day each September 9; and on September 9, 2003, Senator Lisa Murkowski of the state of Alaska proposed similar legislation in the United States Senate. The grassroots movement continues, as more parents and professionals across Canada and around the world use September 9 as the focus date for their awareness campaign strategies.

Ex-Navy and an expert knotter, Brian developed the "FAS Knot"— the wearable symbol of FAS, representing to an international community the re-connecting of Michael Dorris's "Broken Cord." To date, thousands of FAS Knots have been tied and worn in communities from the Canadian Arctic to the southern tip of New Zealand. (Instructions for the FAS Knot are on our website, www.fasworld.com.)

The Tipping Point

We need to declare war on FAS, a war to change attitudes about alcohol abuse, and about stopping alcohol use in pregnancy. This will be costly, and will not depend on posters, or public service pronouncements, nor smug PR gimmicks. It will be to fight for an improvement in housing, a fight for better access to educational opportunities to those who are poor and in minority

groups, a fight for better child care, a fight for better nutrition, and a fight to reduce or eliminate family violence and abuse.
—Dr. Ab Chudley

In his fascinating book, *The Tipping Point: How Little Things Can Make a Big Difference,* Malcolm Gladwell writes that major social changes can occur suddenly, because ideas, messages and behaviour often spread as quickly as epidemics of infectious disease. These "social epidemics" spread mainly by word-of-mouth information.

Tackling FASD requires far more than money. It requires knowledge of the effects of prenatal alcohol, knowledge that reaches from the top levels of government down to individual members of the community. Government departments—health, social services, education and criminal justice—must work together, and plan interlocking policies and programs.

We need national communications programs. Commercials for pharmaceutical products must warn viewers of side effects, so why aren't alcoholic beverage commercials required to warn viewers of the dangers of prenatal alcohol to the fetus?

But government can't do it all. All parts of the community must take responsibility for the permanent damage that is being done to our children before they are born.

Press and TV cover media stars, sports heroes and lascivious politicians at length, and they frequently run items about health issues such as cancer and AIDS. But reporters and editors often feel that because they "did" an item on fetal alcohol five years ago, they are not interested. Unwittingly, they *are* telling stories about FASD every day. Every time they run an item on the homeless, families in poverty, mental illness or a lurid crime, the unmentioned possibility of FASD is there.

Brian and I have met numerous extraordinary people of faith in the past few years, but many regular worshippers prefer to believe that the homeless, the addicted and people in poverty have chosen to live that way. I'd like to see ministers, priests, rabbis and imams encourage their congregations to act with charity and compassion towards the children and adults in their own communities whose intellectual capacities were diminished before they were born.

Business needs to play a larger role. The retail industry loses countless dollars each year because of shoplifting, the common "starter" crime of adolescents with FASD. Insurance agencies pay a fortune to the victims of burglary and car theft, also favourite activities of many young males with FASD. Corporations offering support to organizations working to prevent FASD, or those providing help to alcohol-affected individuals, would be acting out of enlightened self-interest.

Simply telling friends, neighbours and colleagues how FASD affects all of us can have a ripple effect in our own communities. Encouraging students at all levels to take on FASD as a class project can inform future parents about the dangers of alcohol in pregnancy.

Daring to Hope

Eliminating FASD will require large-scale social marketing. Attitudes on drinking and unplanned pregnancy can and must be changed. Teresa Kellerman cites U.S. statistics indicating that about 52 percent of women of childbearing age report the use of alcohol within the past month—and adds that about half of all U.S. pregnancies are unintended. She says that most women who drink will cut down or stop drinking when they learn they are pregnant, but many women do not realize they are pregnant until their second month of pregnancy. These statistics indicate that at least 25 percent of infants are exposed to alcohol during the first trimester, when the fetus is most vulnerable to alcohol. According to Teresa, three groups of pregnant women need prevention education and support. First, heavy drinkers, the alcoholics who may not decrease alcohol use during pregnancy. Second, moderate drinkers who believe the myth that "only women who drink heavily have affected babies"—or whose doctors tell them that "one or two drinks a day won't hurt." Finally, women who are alcohol-affected themselves. They may not be recognized as having a disability, but they have poor judgment and lack impulse control. For these women, prevention education and traditional addiction treatment will likely not be effective. If we don't reach this group, she says, "we are destined to watch the cycle continue with their children and their children's children falling into the ever-widening cracks in the social service system."

Some may feel the challenge is just too big; to them, breaking the cycle of alcohol-damage, poverty and abandonment seems impossible. But people who think this way should remember how effective social marketing has been in changing public attitudes towards cigarette smoking. Since the first U.S. Surgeon-General's report on smoking in 1964, education and public concern about health has radically reduced cigarette use from about 50 percent of American and Canadian adults to around 25 percent.

We have battled countless other major health disasters—and won. The smallpox virus killed as many as 100 million people throughout the centuries, but in 1776 a British country doctor named Edward Jenner invented the principle of vaccination, and two hundred years later, smallpox had been eradicated.

Until the mid-nineteenth century, puerperal or childbed fever was killing about 30 percent of women who gave birth in hospitals. Then a Vienna obstetrician, Ignaz Philipp Semmelweis, observed that women examined by student doctors who had not washed their hands after leaving the autopsy room had high death rates. When doctors began washing their hands with chlorinated lime before examining patients, the death rate in childbirth plummeted.

Few people who were children in the 1940s and 1950s can forget the terrifying polio epidemics that swept North America. Researchers were able to develop a vaccine in the 1950s, and fifty years later, through "Polio Plus," a joint effort of the World Health Organization, Rotary International and the Bill and Melinda Gates Foundation, polio will soon be eradicated worldwide. Brian and I are not alone in hoping that when these three organizations wipe out polio in this decade, they will consider tackling the complex, costly but preventable FASD epidemic that impairs the intelligence of countless numbers of the 133 million babies who come into the world each year.

The Third Generation

A last whirl of the kaleidoscope gave me another view of the complex issue of FASD: my grandchildren are the third generation torn from their biological mothers. I now wonder about their maternal great-grand-mother, an alcoholic who abandoned her daughter, Colette's mother, "Harriet," who later drank through three pregnancies, losing custody of Colette and her two older brothers. Did their great-grandmother have FASD too? We'll never know how far back this cycle goes.

Colette's children have been traumatized by Mummy's emotional distance, and I'm not sure that she can ever parent them full-time again. She was a patient, nurturing mother to her babies, but as preschoolers, eighteen months apart, they are smart, funny—and a handful. While struggling with a power-drunk two-year-old, I'm often amazed that Colette lasted as long as she did. My sense is that for mothers with FASD, parenting is rather like school. They can cope in the first year or two, when the tasks are mainly hands-on and concrete, but the job becomes almost impossible as these little people develop distinct, demanding personalities, and other parental abilites are required, such as empathy, a high tolerance for others' frustrating behaviour and insight into how young children think and feel.

Brian and I are not alone in our new role. Statistics Canada indicates that nearly 40,000 Canadian children under the age of eighteen are living with grandparents. I suspect that FASD may be a root cause in many of these cases: we know several adoptive parents who are raising their children's children, both in our Toronto support group and among online friends.

Only 20 percent of the parents with FASD in Ann Streissguth's secondary disabilities study, and 10 percent of the women with FASD studied by Sterling Clarren were able to raise their children. Jo Nanson has followed mothers with FASD for more than a decade, and says she only knows one who has been a successful parent, and she was helped by tremendous support from a church group. Nanson points out that by not drinking in pregnancy, and ensuring her children are in a secure place, Colette has done the best she can. "In FASD terms, she's a success. Her children have intact brains, and she's made sure they're loved and safe."

Colette currently lives alone in a too-big apartment that was rented for her family of four, and we're trying to figure out how to get out of the lease. Having acquired both a high school diploma and a driver's licence, she's looking for a full-time job working with animals—a job with benefits, so she can go off disability support. She will require a patient employer who understands that she needs much more structure and supervision than the norm.

Cleo, in her mid-twenties, lives with the chronic depression she inherited from her biological parents, plus learning problems (mainly related to math and spatial relationships) and attention deficit disorder (diagnosed when she was eighteen). Her depression is worse in winter, but can be controlled by medication. An excellent caregiver, she spent two years as a personal support worker to a disabled professional in the workplace, and now juggles various clients requiring special care. She is also devoted to her little niece and nephew—although she jokes that as a constant reminder of how difficult it is to be a mother of little kids, they are the best method of birth control. There has been a special young man in her life for some years, but right now she prefers to live alone, cherishing her independence.

Many of our friends—among them two colleagues interviewed for this book—think we're demented for taking on this new challenge. The thought of being in our seventies and raising teenagers *is* terrifying, but there seems to be no workable alternative. We know that if the Children's Aid Society becomes involved we could lose contact with these children forever, and put them at risk of being damaged by a series of foster homes or adoption breakdowns.

Our suburban haven with its tiny bedrooms is all wrong for little kids. Our grandson is occupying our dressing room, our granddaughter the former coat room, and there's no room for Brian's and my clothes in our cramped "master" bedroom. Sometimes I yearn for my empty nest and free time. I often fear I won't have the strength and patience for the next round of advocacy, fighting for children damaged not by prenatal alcohol but by family trauma.

But when we and the kids smush each other together in our morning "huggle," or Brian's inspired goofiness makes them nearly fall off their chairs laughing, or I peek in at those sleeping cherubs at night, I'm grateful to have them in my life, despite the chaos.

We hope that with the next spin of the kaleidoscope, Colette will be able to resume an active and continuing role in her children's lives.

We hope that her commitment to sobriety in pregnancy has given them the mental resilience to survive the current separation.

And when I watch her protective, curly-haired son and his impish little sister nurturing their teddy bears and dolls, I hope that Brian and I will have enough love, health and energy to heal their deep pain, passed down through generations on both sides of their biological families—so that this time around, the cycle of alcoholism and abandonment will truly be broken.

ENDNOTES

1. Ann Streissguth, *Fetal Alcohol Syndrome: A Guide for Families and Communities* (Baltimore: Paul H. Brookes Publishing, 1997), 35.
2. Ibid., 36.
3. See, for example, John W. Olney et al., "Early effects of alcohol exposure," *Science*, 11 February 2000. See also Beena Sood et al., "Prenatal alcohol exposure and childhood behavior at age 6 to 7 years: I. Dose–response effect," *Pediatrics* 108, no. 2 (August 2001), e34.
4. Kathleen Stratton, Cynthia Howe, and Frederick Battaglia, eds., *Fetal Alcohol Syndrome: Diagnosis, Epidemiology, Prevention and Treatment* (Washington, D.C.: Institute of Medicine, National Academy Press, 1996), 77.
5. See, for example, P. D. Sampson, et al, "Incidence of fetal alcohol syndrome and prevalence of alcohol-related neurodevelopmental disorder," *Teratology* 56, no. 5 (November 1997), 317–26; and Ann Streissguth, "Recent Advances in Fetal Alcohol Syndrome and Alcohol Use in Pregnancy," in D. P. Agarwal and Helmut K. Seitz, eds., *Alcohol in Health and Disease* (New York: Marcel Dekker, 2001).
6. Stratton et al., *Fetal Alcohol Syndrome*, 53.
7. Christie Blatchford, "A mother from the depths of hell," *Toronto Sun*, 14 April 1997.
8. Harwood, Henrick J., and Diane M. Napolitano, "Economic Implications of the Fetal Alcohol Syndrome," *Alcohol Health and Research World* (10) (1): 38–43 and 74–75, 1985.

9.   Maureen Weeks, Economic Impact of Fetal Alcohol Syndrome: IR89-100015, report commissioned by State Senator Johne Binkley and presented to Alaska State Legislature, 1989.

10. H. Philip Hepworth, "Jack's Troubled Career: The Costs to Society of a Young Person in Trouble," *National Crime Prevention Strategy* (Canadian government ministry of justice), www.prevention.gc.ca/en/library/publications/economic/jack/index/html.

11. Brenda Cathrine [sic] Stade, "The Burden of Prenatal Exposure to Alcohol: Measurements of Quality of Life and Costs," unpublished Ph.D. thesis, Institute of Medical Science, University of Toronto, 2003.

12. United States Congress, *Consumer Subcommittee on Warning Labels,* Senate Committee on Commerce, Science and Transportation, August 1988.

13. Ann Streissguth, Helen M. Barr, and Paul D. Sampson, "Moderate Prenatal Alcohol Exposure: Effects on Child IQ and Learning Problems at age 7½ years," *Alcoholism Clinical and Experimental Research*, September/October 1990.

14. Olney, et al., "Early effects of alcohol exposure."

15. Jennifer F. Little, interview with author, February 2002.

16. Jennifer F. Little, Peter G. Heppner, and James C. Dornan, "Maternal alcohol consumption during pregnancy and fetal startle behaviour," *Physiology and Behaviour* 76 (2002), 691–94.

17. Dr. Pat Troop, interviewed on "Tonight with Trevor McDonald" (ITV), 28 January 2000, www.independent.co.uk.

18. Royal College of Obstetricians and Gynecologists, "Clinical Green Top Guidelines," *Alcohol Consumption in Pregnancy*, December 1999, www.rcog.org.uk/guidelines.

19. Streissguth, *Fetal Alcohol Syndrome*, 126.

20. Thomas K. Greenfield, "Warning Labels: Evidence of Harm Reduction from Long-term American Surveys," chap. 7 in *Alcohol: Minimising the Harm*, edited by Martin Plant, Eric Single and Tim Stockwell, (London and New York: Free Association Books, 1991), 121.

21. I. Walpole, S. Zubrick, and J. Pontre, "Confounding variables in studying the effects of maternal alcohol consumption before and during pregnancy," *Journal of Epidemiology and Community Health* 43 (1989), 153–61. In 1990 the same researchers published, "Is there a foetal effect with low to moderate use before and during pregnancy?" in *Journal of Epidemiology and Community Health* 44 (1990), 297–301. In 1991 they published "Low to moderate maternal alcohol use before and during pregnancy, and neurobehavioural outcome in the newborn infant," *Developmental Medicine and Child Neurology* 33 (1991), 875–83.

22. Brewers Association of Canada, *Submission to Subcommitee on Bill C-222, An Act to Amend the Food and Drugs Act,* 2 May 1996.

23. New South Wales Department of Neonatal Medicine Protocol Book, www.cs.nsw.gov.au, 3 and 15.

24. C. Guerri, E. Riley, and K. Stromland, "Commentary on the recommendations of the Royal College of Obstetricians and Gynaecologists concerning alcohol consumption in pregnancy," *Alcohol and Alcoholism* 34, no. 4 (1999), 497–501.

25. David N. Whitten, *To Your Health* (New York: HarperCollins West, 1994), 86.

26. Ruth Flanagan, "Man's bizarre 1848 accident leads to study of the brain," *Dallas Morning News*, 14 September 1998.

27. Susan J. Astley, Diane Bailey, Christina Talbot, and Sterling K. Clarren, "Fetal alcohol syndrome (FAS) primary prevention through FAS diagnosis," *Alcohol and Alcoholism* 35, no. 5 (2000). (Two consecutive articles.)

28. See, for example, Olney et al., "Early effects of alcohol exposure," and Stratton et al., *Fetal Alcohol Syndrome,* 165, 166.

29. Kieran O'Malley and Frances M. E. Kapp, *Watch for the Rainbows: True Stories for Educators and Other Caregivers of Children with Fetal Alcohol Spectrum Disorders* (Calgary: Frances Kapp Education, 2001), 11.

30. Streissguth, *Fetal Alcohol Syndrome,* 126–27.

31. Streissguth et al., *Understanding the Occurrence of Secondary Disabilities*, 37.

32. Ibid., 37–41.

33. Royal Canadian Mounted Police website on missing Canadian children: www.ourmissingchildren.ca.

34. Christine Rogan, of the New Zealand government's Alcohol Healthwatch, citing the (now-defunct) *Fetal Alcohol New Zealand Trust Newsletter*, letter to author, spring 2000.

35. Carlos Carcach and Anna Grant, "Imprisonment in Australia: Trends in Prison Populations and Imprisonment Rates, 1982–1998," Australian Institute of Criminology (1999), www.aic.gov.au.

36. Australia National Drug Strategy Household Survey 2001.

37. Ibid.

38. Twenty articles in the *Toronto Star*, from 28 April 1999 to 14 August 1999, and one article on 10 November 2001.

39. National Crime Prevention Strategy website (Ministry of Justice, Canada), www.crime-prevention.org.

40. United States Department of Justice, Bureau of Justice Statistics, www.ojp.usdoj.gov/bjs/eande.htm.

41. United Nations Criminal Justice Information Network (UNCJIN), *Crime and Justice Letter* 2, no. 3, www.uncjin.org.

42. Greg Winter, "California appellate ruling aids foes of 3-strike law," *New York Times*, Dec. 10, 2001.

43. Russell Mokhiber and Robert Weissman, "Sixteen Years for a Snickers Bar," www.commondreams.com, 4 February 2002.

44. *Fetal Alcohol New Zealand Trust,* Newsletter, spring 2000.

45. Harumi Tanaka, "Fetal alcohol syndrome: A Japanese perspective," *Annals of Medicine* 30 (1998), 21–26.

46. Jane Aronson, "Alcohol Related Disorders and Children Adopted from Abroad," www.orphandoctor.com.

47. "Irish among world's biggest boozers, minister says," Reuters, 13 August 2001.

48.   Celia Hall, "Binge drinkers 'risking death,'" (London) *Telegraph*, 12 November 2001.

49.   Donna Debolt, interview with author.

50.   Maggie Brady, *The Health of Young Aborigines,* 1991.

51.   David Square, "Fetal alcohol syndrome epidemic on Manitoba reserve," *Canadian Medical Association Journal* 157 (1 July 1997), 59–60.

52.   Statistics Canada, births and birth rate, www.statscan.ca.

53.   United States National Center for Health Statistics, www.cdc.gov/nchs/rclcases/.

54.   Streissguth et al., *Understanding the Occurrence of Secondary Disabilities,* 5.

BIBLIOGRAPHY

Books and Reports

Boland, Fred J., Rebecca Burrill, Michelle Duwyn, and Jennifer Karp. *Fetal Alcohol Syndrome: Implications for Correctional Service.* Ottawa: Research Branch of Correctional Service Canada, 1996. Well-written overview of FASD in Canada's justice system. Out of print at press time. Available online at www.csc.scc.gc.ca.

Brady, Maggie, *The Health of Young Aborigines aged 12 to 25.* Published by the [Australian] National Clearinghouse for Youth Studies for the National Youth Affairs Research Scheme, Canberra 1992. Report indicates the striking similarity in alcohol-related problems of Australian and North American youth of indigenous background.

Conry, Julianne, and Diane K. Fast, M.D. *Fetal Alcohol Syndrome and the Criminal Justice System.* Vancouver: Law Foundation of British Columbia and B.C. Fetal Alcohol Syndrome Resource Society, 2000. Contains case studies of individuals with FASD; explains why the criminal justice system fails to serve their needs or prevent them from committing further crimes. Available from B.C. FAS Resource Society, P.O. Box 525, Maple Ridge, BC V2X 3P2. Telephone (604) 467 7101. Another must for criminal-justice professionals.

Conry, Julianne, Diane K. Fast, Christine A. Loock, "Youth in the Criminal Justice System: Identifying FAS and Other Alcohol-Related Neurodevelopmental Disabilities," B.C. Fetal Alcohol Syndrome Resource Society, March, 1997.

Greenfield, Thomas K. "Warning Labels: Evidence on Harm Reduction from Long-term American Surveys." Chap. 7 in *Alcohol: Minimising the Harm*, eds. Martin Plant, Eric Single, and Tim Stockwell. London and New York: Free Association Books, 1999.

Indian and Northern Affairs Canada, Royal Commission on Aboriginal Peoples, *Gathering Strength: Report of the Royal Commission on Aboriginal Peoples.* Published by the Minister of Public Works and Government Services, 1996. A massive, comprehensive investigation of the destructive effects of the European immigration and twentieth century industrialization on the lives of indigenous North Americans.

Kleinfeld, Judith, and Siobhan Westcott, eds. *Fantastic Antone Succeeds.* Fairbanks: University of Alaska Press, 1993. Positive book with dozens of strategies developed by parents and professionals living or working with children with FASD.

Kleinfeld, Judith, Siobhan Westcott, and Barbara Morse, eds. *Fantastic Antone Grows Up*, Fairbanks: University of Alaska Press, 2000. The editors try their best to be positive, but the prognosis for many adolescents and young adults with FASD seems bleak.

Malbin, Diane. *Fetal Alcohol Syndrome/Fetal Alcohol Effects: Strategies for Professionals.* Center City, MN: Hazelden, 1993. Malbin, birth mother of a child with FASD, outlines the "paradigm shift" in thinking that professionals and families must undergo in dealing with youngsters with FASD: "they can not" rather than "they will not." A thirty-nine-page gem.

Miller, Jerome G. *Search and Destroy: African-American Males in the Criminal Justice System*, Cambridge University Press, 1996. Meticulous research regarding systemic racism in the U.S. justice system.

Mountford, Allan. *'Cause It's Not My Fault.* Self-published. Excellent
    handbook for educators of adolescents with FAS, by special
    education teacher Mountford, based on his M.Ed. thesis.
    Contact him at 106 Coleman Crescent, Janetville, ON L0B 1K0, or at
    <Mountford_Allan@durham.edu.on.ca>.

O'Malley, Kieran, and Frances M. E. Kapp. *Watch for the Rainbows: True
    Stories for Educators and Other Caregivers of Children with Fetal
    Alcohol Spectrum Disorders.* Calgary: Frances Kapp Education, 2001.
    A warm and positive look at the strengths of alcohol-affected
    children.

Stratton, Kathleen, Cynthia Howe, and Frederick Battaglia, eds. *Fetal Alcohol
    Syndrome: Diagnosis, Epidemiology and Treatment.* Washington,
    D.C.: Institute of Medicine, National Academy Press, 1996.
    Thorough, basic medical textbook on the effects of alcohol on the
    developing fetus, and how these disabilities impact on the individ-
    ual and society.

Streissguth, Ann. *Fetal Alcohol Syndrome: A Guide for Families and
    Communities.* Baltimore, MD: Paul H. Brookes Publishing, 1997.
    Highly recommended, fascinating and positive book, by the world's
    leading researcher in the psychological effects of FASD.

———. "Recent Advances in Fetal Alcohol Syndrome and Alcohol Use in
    Pregnancy." In *Alcohol in Health and Disease*, D. P. Agarwal, and
    Helmut K. Seitz, eds. New York: Marcel Dekker, Inc., 2001.

Streissguth, Ann, Helen M. Barr, Julia Kogan, and Fred L. Bookstein.
    *Understanding the Occurrence of Secondary Disabilities in Clients with
    Fetal Alcohol Syndrome (FAS) and Fetal Alcohol Effects (FAE).* Seattle:
    University of Washington School of Medicine, Fetal Alcohol and
    Drug Unit, 1996. A ground-breaking study on long-term outcomes
    of individuals with prenatal alcohol damage. Only seventy-one
    pages, mostly easy-to-read graphs. A *must* for parents and profes-
    sionals. Send a US$5 money order to University of Washington, Fetal
    Alcohol and Drug Unit, 180 Nickerson, Suite 309, Seattle, WA 98109.

Streissguth, Ann, and Jonathan Kanter, eds. *The Challenge of Fetal Alcohol Syndrome: Overcoming Secondary Disabilities.* Seattle: University of Washington Press, 1997. Collection of twenty-two articles from international researchers, presented at an international conference at the University of Washington in 1997.

Szabo, Paul. *FAS: The Real Brain Drain.* Self-published by a Liberal MP. Telephone (905) 822 2111 or (613) 992 4848. A good, free, basic primer on FASD.

Research Papers and Medical/Scientific Journals

Astley, Susan J., Diane Bailey, Christina Talbot, and Sterling K. Clarren. "Fetal alcohol syndrome (FAS) primary prevention through FAS diagnosis." *Alcohol and Alcoholism* 35, no. 5 (2000). Two consecutive articles.

Brewers Association of Canada, *Submission to Subcommittee on Bill C-222, An Act to Amend the Food and Drugs Act,* 2 May 1996.

Debolt, Donna and Mary Berube. "Guidelines for Intervention with Families." Unpublished report used in training sessions by two social workers specializing in FASD. More information available from Donna Debolt: <Donna.Debolt@gov.ab.ca>.

Guerri, Consuelo, Kerstin Stromland, and Edward Riley. "Commentary on the recommendations of the Royal College of Obstetricians and Gynaecologists concerning alcohol consumption in pregnancy." *Alcohol and Alcoholism* 34, no. 4 (1999), 497–501.

Harwood, Henrick J. and Diane M. Napolitano, "Economic Implications of the Fetal Alcohol Syndrome," *Alcohol Health and Research World* 10(1): 38–43 and 74–75 , 1985. 20-year-old look at financial costs to society of U.S. individuals with full fetal alcohol syndrome.

Hayes, Lorian, "Grog Babies." Fascinating unpublished academic paper explores the levels of community knowledge relating to "Foetal Alcohol Syndrome" and attitudes of young women and men towards alcohol and pregnancy in two Aboriginal communities in Queensland, Australia.

Little, Jennifer F., Peter G. Heppner, and James C. Dornan. "Maternal alcohol consumption during pregnancy and fetal startle behaviour." *Physiology and Behaviour* 76 (2002), 691–94.

Loop, Karen Q., and Mary D. Nettleman, M.D. "Obstetrical textbooks: Recommendations about drinking during pregnancy." *American Journal of Preventive Medicine* 23, no. 1 (2002): 136–38.

Olney, John W. et al. "Ethanol-induced apoptotic neurodegeneration and fetal alcohol syndrome." *Science*, 11 February 2000. Cited in an article by Paul Recer,, "Link found between alcohol and brain cell death in young," Associated Press, 10 February 2000.

Sampson, P. D., Ann Streissguth, R. E. Little, S. K. Clarren, P. Dehaene, J. W. Hanson, and J. M. Graham, Jr. "Incidence of fetal alcohol syndrome and prevalence of alcohol-related neurodevelopmental disorder." *Teratology* 56, no. 5 (November 1997).

Sood, Beena, M.D., Virginia Delaney-Black, M.D., Chandice Covington, Beth Nordstrom-Klee, Joel Ager, Thomas Templin, James Janisse, Susan Martier, and Robert J. Sokol, M.D. "Prenatal alcohol exposure and childhood behavior at age 6 to 7 years: i. Dose–response effect." *Pediatrics* 108, no. 2 (August 2001).

Square, David. "Fetal alcohol syndrome epidemic on Manitoba reserve." *Canadian Medical Association Journal* 157 (1 July 1997), 59–60.

Streissguth, Ann, Helen M. Barr, and Paul D. Sampson. "Moderate prenatal alcohol exposure: Effects on child IQ and learning problems at age 7½ years." *Alcoholism Clinical and Experimental Research* (September/October 1990).

Tanaka, Harumi, M.D. "Fetal alcohol syndrome: A Japanese perspective." *Annals of Medicine* 30 (1998): 21–26.

United States Congress, Senate Committee on Commerce, Science and Transportation. *Consumer Subcommittee on Warning Labels,* August 1988.

Walpole, I., S. Zubrick, and J. Pontre. "Confounding variables in studying the effects of maternal alcohol consumption before and during pregnancy." *Journal of Epidemiology and Community Health* 43 (1989), 153–61.

———. "Is there a foetal effect with low to moderate use before and during pregnancy?" *Journal of Epidemiology and Community Health* 44 (1990), 297–301.

———. "Low to moderate maternal alcohol use before and during pregnancy, and neurobehavioural outcome in the newborn infant," *Developmental Medicine and Child Neurology* 33 (1991): 875–83.

Newspapers and Newsletters

Blatchford, Christie. "A mother from the depths of hell." *Toronto Sun,* 4 April 1997.

Flanagan, Ruth. "Man's bizarre 1848 accident leads to study of the brain." *Dallas Morning News,* 14 September 1998.

Fetal Alcohol New Zealand Trust, Newsletter, Spring 2000.

Gailus, Jeff. "Who killed Garrett Campiou?" *Alberta Views,* May/June 2001.

Hall, Celia. "Binge drinkers 'risking death.'" *London Telegraph,* 12 November 2001.

"Irish among world's biggest boozers, minister says." Reuters, 13 August 2001.

Toronto Star, twenty articles following the trial of John Paul Roby and his eventual death. 28 April 1999 to 14 August 1999, and 10 November 2001.

Websites

AFCARS Report (Administration on Children, Youth and Families), www.acf.dhhs.gov/programs/cb.

Aronson, Jane, M.D. "Alcohol Related Disorders and Children Adopted from Abroad," www.orphandoctor.com.

Australia National Drug Strategy Household Survey 2001, www.nationaldrugstrategy.gov.au

Carcach, Carlos, and Anna Grant. "Imprisonment in Australia: Trends in Prison Populations and Imprisonment Rates, 1982–1998." Australian Institute of Criminology, 1999, www.aic.gov.au.

Mokhiber, Russell, and Robert Weissman. "Sixteen Years for a Snickers Bar," www.commondreams.com, 4 February 2002.

Ministry of Justice (Canada). *National Crime Prevention Strategy*, www.prevention.org.

New South Wales Department of Neonatal Medicine Protocol Book, www.cs.nsw.gov.au.

North America Council on Adoptable Children, www.nacac.org.

Royal College of Obstetricians and Gynaecologists. "Clinical Green Top Guidelines," *Alcohol Consumption in Pregnancy* (December 1999), www.rcog.org.uk/guidelines.

Royal Canadian Mounted Police website on missing Canadian children, www.ourmissingchildren.ca.

Statistics Canada, births and birth rate, www.statscan.ca.

United Nations Criminal Justice Information Network (UNCJIN), *Crime and Justice Letter* 2, no. 3, www.uncjin.org.

United States Department of Justice, Bureau of Justice Statistics, www.ojp.usdoj.gov/bjs/cacdc.htm.

United States National Center for Health Statistics, www.cdc/nchs/releases/.

OTHER RESOURCES

Recommended Books

Cook, Paula, Richard Kellie, Kathy Jones, and Laura Goosen. *Tough Kids and Substance Abuse.* Winnipeg: Addictions Foundation of Manitoba Library, 2000. Designed to be photocopied, a series of easy lessons for difficult adolescents, plus how-to's for teachers and other professionals who deal with these kids.

Dorris, Michael. *The Broken Cord.* New York: HarperCollins, 1989. Award-winning, heartbreaking memoir by the adoptive father of a young native American boy.

Dorris, Michael. *Paper Trail.* New York: HarperCollins, 1994. A collection of essays, containing some well-written reflections on fetal alcohol syndrome and fetal alcohol effects.

Graaefe, Sara. *Parenting Children Affected by FASD: A Guide for Daily Living.* Vancouver: Society of Special Needs Adoptive Parents (SNAP), revised 2003. An excellent guide for both families and professionals.

Kranowitz, Carol Stock. *The Out-of-Sync Child: Recognizing and Coping with Sensory Integration Dysfunction.* New York: Perigee, 2001. Many children with FASD also have SI dysfunction, a problem with the central nervous system that causes them to be oversensitive or undersensitive to touch, taste, smell, sound or sight.

Kulp, Jodee. *Our FAScinating Journey: The Best We Can Be.* An adoptive mother in Minnesota develops a program of nutrition, physical training and brain-development exercises to boost her alcohol-affected daughter's learning ability. Available from Better Endings, New Beginnings, 6289 Brunswick Avenue N., Brooklyn Park, MN 55429, (763) 531 9548, www.betterendings.org.

Lasser, Peggy. *Challenges and Opportunities: A Handbook for Teachers of Students with Special Needs with a Focus on Fetal Alcohol Syndrome.* Vancouver School Board, 1999. An excellent book, outlining strategies for anyone working with youngsters for FASD.

Nasdijj. *Blood Runs like a River through My Dreams.* New York: Houghton Mifflin, 2000. Luminous poetic essays by a writer of half-aboriginal, half-Caucasian origin living in the U.S. Southwest, who adopted a small Native American boy with fetal alcohol syndrome.

Video

Different Directions. Three excellent 23-minute videos produced by Toronto's Canadian Mothercraft/Breaking the Cycle and Ontario's North for the Children. Health Canada, $50. Call Canadian Mothercraft for more information: (416) 920 5983.

Some Suggested FASD Websites

www.fasworld.com. Contains many links, contacts and other info, particularly relating to International FAS Awareness Day, held each September 9 by volunteers in many communities across Canada and the U.S., and in Germany, Poland, Luxembourg, Sweden, Croatia, South Africa, Australia and New Zealand.

www.fasstar.com. An enormous, constantly updated site containing numerous articles and links, operated by FASDay co-founder Teresa Kellerman of the FAS Family Resource Center of Tucson, Arizona. Teresa also operates www.fasday.com, offering advice and suggestions for people planning FASDay events.

www.ccsa.ca. This site for the Canadian Centre for Substance Abuse, funded by Health Canada and the Brewers Association of Canada, contains many journal articles and lists resources such as support organizations and diagnostic clinics. The information hotline number is (800) 559 4514, and resource personnel will mail additional material on request.

www.acbr.com. A Canadian site that will get you onto FASlink, the international online support group. It is also your access route to the FASlink archives, where you will find answers to many questions. You can also get onto FASlink by e-mailing <majordomo@listserv.rivernet.net> with the message "subscribe FASlink."

depts.washington.edu/fadu/. Another frequently updated site. Contains many articles by Professor Ann Streissguth and others at the University of Washington Faculty of Medicine in Seattle. It also contains links to family support groups and professionals in the U.S., Canada and worldwide, plus a list of newsletters and other publications dealing with FASD.

www.arbi.org. An Alberta site with much valuable information and many links.

home.golden.net/~fasat. Operated by Fetal Alcohol Support Awareness and Training (FASAT) in Guelph, Ontario.

Buying books online

Books on FASD can be purchased through www.chapters.indigo.ca, www.amazon.ca and a few specialty bookstores with online outlets, such as FAS Bookshelf in Vancouver (www.fasbookshelf.com), and Parentbooks in Toronto (www.parentbookstore.com). The University of Saskatchewan bookstore (www.uofsbookstore.com) has an enormous FASD section, with several hundred academic titles relating to addiction, brain injury, psychology and aboriginal issues.

INDEX

aboriginal communities, FASD and, 48–49, 205–7, 223–25, 236

abuse. *See* emotional abuse; physical abuse; sexual abuse and assault(s)

the Achenbach test, 33

acting-out behaviour (teenage), 23–24, 100–103, 178–81, 183–84, 195–96

Adam (Lynn Frank's adoptive son with FASD), 158–60, 171–72

ADHD. *See* attention deficit hyperactivity disorder

adoption(s)

breakdown(s) of, 50, 160, 163, 171

discussions with the children about, 16

successful prescreening for FASD and, 111–13, 172–74, 238–42, 245–59, 267

the urgent need for more, 266–68

Adoption Council of Canada, 161

Adoption Disclosure Register (Ontario), 66

aggressive behaviours. *See also* sensory processing overload

prenatal alcohol exposure and, 85, 158–60, 164, 170, 229, 246

AIDS, 13, 235–36

Alateen, 123

alcohol. *See also* pregnancy, risks from alcohol during; taxes

addictive nature of, 134

cross-addictions and, 28

cultural encouragement for consuming, 152

dose-dependent effects of, 80

historic notes of risks from, 42

manuals on pregnancy and, 87–88

measurement units of, 84–85

medical attitudes and tolerance toward, 87–88

parental usage of, 51–52

payments made in, 235

predispositions to use given FASD, 102

public tolerance and carelessness concerning, 133–35

teratogenic nature of, 46, 80, 88

toxicity to fetal cells of, 86

alcoholic beverage industry, lobbying by, 91

alcohol-related neurodevelopmental disorder (ARND). *See also* FAE; FASD

defined, 45–46

long term outcome from, 47

Alejandro, Mercedes (mother of Nicholas, young adult with FASD), 97, 135–36

BONNIE BUXTON is a journalist who has written articles for numerous Canadian magazines and newspapers. She and her husband, Brian Philcox, are co-founders of FASworld Canada (www.FASworld.com), the Canadian nonprofit organization that works at building awareness, and co-founders of International FAS Awareness Day, observed by volunteers across North America and many other countries. A native Albertan, she lives in Toronto.

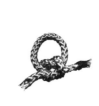